Diary of a H.O.
(House Officer)

A collection of short stories from a
surgeon's first year of training

Dr. Brandon Green

Copyright

ACKNOWLEDGEMENTS

I would like to thank my wife and children for their support, as without them this book would have been finished a couple years ago.

Two of my favorite surgeon sayings apply to this book,

"It's better to be lucky than good."

"The enemy of good, is better."

DISCLAIMER

This book contains real short stories from an intern year, which is the first year of hospital-based training after graduating from medical school. The book follows an intern class, of three new Doctors, on their journey of survival and education in a surgery training program. The included short stories, or some variation of the stories, are likely playing out at your local hospital as you read this information.

Including but not limited to the names, characters, locations, incidents, brands, advice, dates/times, hospital and surgery information/protocols, and so forth in this book are provided for entertainment purposes only and are done so with anonymity and without any public disclosure of identifiable information. Patient, physician, staff, and other names have been changed. Although the stories are true, changes have been made to ensure patient privacy including following HIPPA protocols and hospital privacy and indemnity.

The book details the author's personal experiences in regards to surgery intern year training. The author is not your healthcare provider. The author and the publisher are providing this book and its contents on an "as is" basis and make no representations or warranties of any kind with respect to this book and its contents. The author and the publisher disclaim all such representations and warranties, do not use this book for medical advice. The author and publisher do not represent or warrant that the information accessible via this book is accurate, complete, or current. Medical advice should come from a reader's own in person independent physician-patient relationship.

The statements made about any products or services have not been reviewed by the US Food and Drug Administration. They are not meant to diagnose, treat, cure, or prevent any condition or disease. Reader discretion is advised, mature audience only. The book is listed for adult audiences only and is not marketed to underage individuals. Throughout the book there are opinions and occurrences which are not the direct opinion of the author or physicians and surgeons in general. The content is not suitable for minors.

Neither the author, publisher, hospital or healthcare system nor any contributors, editors, or other representatives will be liable for the damages arising out of or in connection with this literary work. This is a comprehensive limitation of liability that applies to all damages of any kind including (without limitation) compensatory; direct or indirect or consequential damages, loss of data, income or profit; loss of or damage to property and claims of third parties. The author has taken necessary and appropriate steps to ensure anonymity of themselves as well as the patients, practice, hospital, medical board, and certification board the author is involved with. Under no circumstances will the author be liable for this information as pertains to professional practice, licensing, board certification, hospital credentialing, and any other reasonably necessary to practice medicine and surgery; and you consent to read by proceeding,

You understand this book is not intended as a substitute for consultation with a licensed healthcare practitioner. This book provides content related to physical and/or mental health issues. As such, use of this book implies acceptance of this disclaimer.

Thank you for reading the legal statement. Now take a deep breath, buckle up, and prepare for a wild adventure into modern healthcare and society!

CONTENTS

FORWARD

I'm impressed not only with the content of this book but also with the author remaining anonymous and donating a portion of the profits to medical charities. Regardless of whether you're in medical training right now, you trained 40 years ago, or you have nothing to do with healthcare, this is an accurate portrayal of daily life in the hospital. We're all humans, regardless of whether you are the patient or the doctor, and life is a roller-coaster ride of mental and physical changes. This is an honest look at the state of society and healthcare in the 21st century, and it's a breath of fresh air during the time of political correctness and cancel culture in our society.

These brilliant, dedicated, caring interns that have worked hard academically and have been at the top of their class for at least 21 years of education are thrown from medical school graduation into the intern year—known as the most grueling year, both professionally and personally—as they put that knowledge and resolve to the test and start to work in the public sector. Some of these interns have spent those 21 years in a library at elite schools with other highly educated and motivated people; now they are thrown into a downtown emergency department with little to no instruction on how to communicate with regular people that come in for help.

Can you imagine giving up the best decade of your life (by most accounts)—your 20s—to this education and training, to be saddled with debt and a healthcare system within which the doctor is losing autonomy and is disrespected by patients and the administration? Somehow interns must navigate this and learn to do what's right for patients. No wonder there are fewer applicants for medical school than any other time, and if admission standards are dropped, what does that do for you and your family's health in the future?

I truly believe that this book may save your life and shed light on the fluid healthcare situation in the United States of America, and that it may perhaps enact change in the future.

Best health and happiness,

Anonymous MD

Board Certified Trauma Surgeon (over 30 years' experience)

INTRODUCTION

It was a bright, sunny day at the end of June when three lives came together, embarking on a journey that would change each of their lives and the world around them forever. Years of education and training had prepared them for the "real world" where they would no longer be students but resident physicians. They were to be thrown from a world of academic elites and socialites into a Level 1 trauma center in a poverty-stricken, large, downtown city hospital.

David was a true country bumpkin, a southern gentleman who was naïve and hardworking, bred from a generation of farming turned heating-and-cooling workers after the turn of the century. A guy who carried a gun at all times, David would go home to hunt wild boars, and he never turned down work. The oldest of five children, he was the star and led his siblings by example. Pushed by his family, he ended up in medical school with plans to give back to the less fortunate in the South. Now he was thrown into a large East Coast city, which was pretty amazing for someone who was taught in school that the Civil War was called the War of Northern Aggression.

Samantha was from the Midwest and appeared to have it all. She could charm an individual or hold an audience of 100 on the edge of their seat. She got a B in the third grade, and that really pissed her off. She never got a B again, and she graduated as valedictorian of her high school, her large state university, and medical school—not to mention she was an all-conference athlete in college. The ultimate extrovert, bubbly and energetic, Samantha had won "most likely to achieve" and "funniest" at multiple levels, but she was exhausted at the end of the day.

Robert was raised by a single mother in the inner city and was more worldly than book smart. High school (which he barely passed) was plagued with clear bookbags, a lottery system for a locker, and metal detectors. He'd had an armed policeman in his schools since he was in kindergarten, not to protect kids but to keep people from the streets out. Robert went to college on a whim with an athletic scholarship and almost went home the first month there. He got a 9 out of 100 on his first college biology exam and went to student services asking for help. Mentors influenced him along the way, and somehow he made it through medical school.

These three had made it into one of the most sought-after surgery training programs in the country. They didn't lack confidence. However, everything they thought they knew was about to change, and they would have to find new confidence in themselves to continue and survive. For numerous years they were told that one person in each class had quit or been fired, and to look at the three of them, the director and the hospital planned to graduate only two of them. They bonded over this and were determined to be the first class to graduate all of them.

Orientation started out well. They received a large packet of papers, a hospital tour, and their ID badge, pager, and schedule. The chief surgery resident spent a few hours with them, talking down to them and belittling them, preparing them for the next several years' journey.

One rotation on the schedule was feared the most by the new intern resident; it's affectionately called H.O. or house officer. This was the rotation that would make or break you, as it would essentially cram as much patient experience into as small amount of time as possible. Every hospital training program has this rotation. You expect to ignore duty hour restrictions and work for approximately 20 hours per day and not talk to your family. On average, residents lose between 15 and 20 pounds during this four-week block. Essentially the 10,000 hours required to become an expert are crammed into these blocks through training years. When your doctor says, "I've seen this once before ..." or "One time in training ...," they likely saw whatever the condition is on the house officer rotation.

Next, David, Samantha, and Robert met with the director of the program, a 50-something hotshot surgeon who wasn't told no enough growing up—the kind of surgeon who thinks he doesn't have to communicate with patients and families, who takes steroids (and often recreational drugs), and who is paid well and lives in a luxury home. He's now on his third wife, who is a trophy. He spent 20 minutes yelling at David, Samantha, and Robert, stating they would only do 80 hours a week on logs, never file a complaint with the program, protect attendings first, and care for patients second. He said he was going to fire one of them, so who was it going to be? You know when you're on for the house, you will make the most mistakes. These mistakes could cost patients' lives, but most importantly they could cost you your career.

The house officer pager was given to Robert, and his rotation block began. The pager went off, blaring, and Robert gasped, jumping up, excited and naïve regarding his first page. On the other end of the phone, they want to talk to the doctor, so he looks around ... and realizes it's him.

CHAPTER 1
Lightbulb Idea

The surgeons' lounge is a separate area, kind of a traditional sanctuary for surgeons. Nurses and sales representatives are not allowed access, and even nurse practitioners and physician assistants are not typically allowed in. The conversations in the lounge—about hospital and personal business—are real and funny. Residents are allowed into the lounge, but the short supply of computers means they must defer to attendings.

Robert was on weekend house officer shift and walking through the surgeons' lounge when the general surgeon on call, Dr. Foster, said, "Look at this asshole, Robert!" Foster was a younger, hotshot general surgeon who said what was on his mind without filtering it or thinking first. "Literally, Robert, look at this asshole."

"What do you mean?" Robert replied, at which time the X-rays popped up on the screen showing the rectum and intestinal tract. Deep to the sphincter was a sizeable lightbulb that appeared intact, having not broken in the rectum.

"Look! An enlightening asshole!" shouted Dr. Foster.

Robert went to the OR, operating room, with Dr. Foster, and the patient (who obviously had either psychiatric issues or recreational issues) was wheeled into the OR and placed on the operating table as anesthesia was started. Dr. Foster reported the patient was a frequent flyer—someone who commonly comes to the ER (emergency room) with complaints and wants to spend several days at the hospital, even if that's under a psychiatric hold.

Once the anesthesia took hold, the sphincter tone relaxed entirely, and the lightbulb simply slid right out of the patient's rectum and anus, completely intact and undamaged. Dr. Foster was elated and asked Robert to fill out the paperwork for patient to be discharged from the recovery unit. Surgery took about 30 seconds. There was no incision, and the patient could go home that day as long as anesthesia was okay with it.

The patient did well with recovery and was asked to leave. He refused. Security was called, and the patient was forced to leave, yelling out, "I'll be back," while laughing.

Robert is still puzzled about why people want to stay in the hospital. What does it say about current society if a patient's home life is so bad that they want to be in the hospital or a psychiatric ward instead of home?

As expected, about three hours later Robert was paged and asked to meet the on-call urologist at the ER. He knew exactly which patient this was even before being told the patient's name or looking up the patient's information in the computer, and he ran down to the ER.

Dr. Garbarski, a seasoned, award-winning urologist with about 34 years in practice, was down at the ER bay, staring at the X-ray monitor. "Robert, you're not going to believe this, but ..."

Robert turned to the monitor, and all he could think about was pain. The X-rays showed the man had placed two AAA batteries in his urethra, the hole in the penis where urine and semen exit. He returned because he was having trouble urinating.

On physical exam, they discovered tearing of the soft tissues at the head of this man's penis. Robert had to insert a supra pubic catheter to drain the bladder and try to decrease the risk of infection and complications.

The patient was admitted to the hospital, and Dr. Garbarski and Robert extracted the batteries in the OR. This was a multi-hour case, and it was painful to be involved. After a couple hours spent removing the batteries and repairing the penis, the patient was sent to recovery and post-op.

In the end, the patient got what he was after—or so we think. He got to stay at the hospital. He was "pink slipped," which means he was sent to the psychiatric ward and held there until the hospital and physician team felt it was okay to release him. The patient might need an inpatient stay in the psychiatric unit and some form of rehab.

Dr Garbarski—and even Robert, the resident intern—had seen a lot of body-mutilation issues over the years, but this was the worst experience during their intern year, even above tales of patients swallowing nails or other materials, clamping sexual organs, and putting hamsters in the anus and lighting the hamsters on fire. Although the anus is the most common cavity from which foreign objects need to be dislodged, this was the most bizarre, painful situation Robert encountered during his intern year.

CHAPTER 2
High Five

Samantha grew up in rural Illinois, the daughter of two factory workers, and she was the smartest, most motivated person any of the other residents had ever met. She was the kind of smart that's brash and appealing. She had a quick wit and was outspoken. She had "it," and "it" was book smarts and the strongest work ethic of any incoming resident.

As house officer, a surgical resident takes care of both the house and unassigned patients—the patients that either don't have insurance or don't have a primary care physician and who are not advantageous enough for the hospital to take on, meaning no or minimal payment to the hospital. Essentially this breaks down to community service and resident training.

Samantha was assigned a new patient who came in with flu-like symptoms. The initial work-up was for pneumonia; however, labs quickly showed a much more devastating process. Her HIV was positive, and her CD4 count was one of the lowest ever seen at our Level 1 trauma center. In other words, she had AIDS, which was not listed in her medical history. Samantha's attending was a nephrologist, Dr. Smith, who had been written up numerous times for poor bedside manner.

For the first time, the two of them had to tell a patient that not only was she HIV positive, but also that she had AIDS. Samantha asked Dr. Smith if she could lead the bedside conversation because she didn't want his rough-and-tough style to break this news to her patient. Thankfully he agreed.

When they walked into the room, the patient was difficult to awaken. She had matted hair and appeared unkempt. The years had been rough on her. At only 50 years old, she appeared well into her 80s. Years of stress and street living had taken its toll on this patient. She was combative and didn't trust anyone.

Samantha pulled two chairs over and sat beside the patient, making direct eye contact—everything she was taught to do to set the stage for this announcement.

The patient, Ms. Thomas, said, "Well, get on with it. What's going on?"

Samantha replied, "Your blood tests have come back positive for HIV, and we think you're dying of AIDS."

Ms. Thomas said, "HIV? Nah, that's nothing. They told me I had that in the mid-1980s." She must have seen the stunned looks on the doctors' faces because Ms. Thomas added, "What? They told me mine wasn't bad then, so I didn't worry about it." (This means the patient had lived at least the past 30 years with no treatment!)

"Wait a second," Ms. Thomas said. "I bet this is why my ex-husband and his new wife hate me. Could this be why a lot of my boyfriends and lovers over the past 30 years have died? I just thought they all didn't like my personality and that their deaths were bad luck."

For the first time in her life, Samantha was speechless. She realized the more she tried to explain HIV and AIDS, the less the patient understood and paid attention. Then there was an ethical dilemma: Should they treat this patient and get her well enough to be discharged, knowing she was likely not going to take care of herself and could put others at risk? Treatment went well, and she was eventually sent home.

The infectious disease specialist worked with the patient and a local university-based, large hospital to study her. (Infectious disease specialists are typically academics who manage antibiotics and antivirals, the kind of doctors who spend minimal time talking to patients and significant time working in the chart and finding the right combinations of medications to treat complex diseases. Look for them in the hospital; for some reason—perhaps as part of their training or to decrease bacteria risk—they typically wear bow ties.)

The specialist and the hospital wanted to know how her immune system could have sustained for as long as it did with HIV. The patient was lost to follow-up and never came back for an appointment. She could have been studied with some genetic testing and possibly saved millions of lives.

CHAPTER 3
Tricks and Ex Fix

Samantha was in the middle of a grueling 30-hour shift when she got a chance to go to the call room, which was (at least at our center, and most centers I visited) just below a dormitory when it came to cleanliness and accommodations. There were separate male and female bathrooms, a fridge containing stale food, one old pool table that leaned, a white board on which were written all the records of lab values at the hospital over the past few years (for example a Hemoglobin A1c of 21.5 which is a diabetic marker of 3 months of an approximately 570 blood sugar), and about 12 individual rooms containing a bed, a chair, and a computer, and with luck, a working television. The speaker in the room called out whole hospital calls, as well as overhead pages.

Samantha grabbed new linens from the cupboard, made the bed, and laid down, exhausted, in her white coat and supplies and promptly passed out asleep. This was the kind of deep sleep residents get, and if you've been through training, you understand. It's a sort of awake-but-asleep state where you hit deep REM sleep almost immediately after closing your eyes. It's sort of a constant dream state, and you're not able to tell the difference between being awake and asleep. This is why residents do not want to sleep and mix their sleep and wake cycles; it can cause them (potentially) to make mistakes with patient care. When someone looks at you and says, "Wow, you look like a zombie!" that's a good comparison to this state residents can find themselves in.

Right after falling asleep, Samantha's pager blared through the room. She was groggy when she called, and the ER said there was a Level 1 trauma. They needed her to come down for an orthopedic evaluation of a patient in the trauma bay. Samantha thought she was dreaming, but she headed to the ER.

The trauma bay is where all patients are brought immediately for either Level 1 or Level 2 traumas. EMS or police dispatch calls and says they are en route with a high-risk patient, and all teams assemble within about three to five minutes. (It's actually quite impressive if you ever get to experience it in person.) The teams know their role, everyone reviews the brief information they have before the patient arrives, the lead determines the level of trauma, and everyone performs their role. This is efficient at the same time that it's chaotic. A common occurrence is when a multi-vehicle crash occurs and multiple people come into the trauma bay at once, all clinging to life, and the team starts working. Falls from heights, crush injuries, gunshot wounds, knife wounds, blunt-force injuries, and failed suicide attempts are also common Level 1 and Level 2 traumas.

Samantha met the orthopedic trauma fellow, and he told her to assemble supplies. The patient had multiple injuries, but the biggest issue was a pelvic fracture. There are some vital issues with pelvic fractures: They can lead to lifelong pain and deformity with walking, but a bigger risk is that the bladder and rectum can be involved. If they are, they can spill their contents into the body, creating a high risk for infection, complications, and loss of life.

The EMS brought in the 20-year-old, 98-pound, Caucasian woman whose pink wig was pulled half off her blonde hair, not woven into her hair. She was in tall, high-heeled boots, her fishnet stockings came only to her mid-thigh, and she was wearing only panties and a buttoned blazer. She had a cell phone, a lot of cash, a small amount of crack cocaine, and condoms with her at the scene—no other belongings. She was found sitting in the street after being hit by a car; the driver left the scene.

Samantha quickly began the orthopedic full-body survey. Typically, general surgery does the survey as well. As in every other trauma, the tech cuts off all the patient's clothes, and the person then lies there naked in a large tray on a table. The team looks for injuries and documents their findings, the respiratory team secures breathing, large-bore IV lines are placed for access, and antibiotics and other sedative drugs are started. This large team of people examine every inch of the person and all their orifices in order to catch additional injuries. X-rays of the whole body are performed on-site.

Once that is all done, the patient is stabilized and then sent for imaging, surgery, or further ER work-up, and their next of kin is contacted.

Fortunately, in this case, the patient's bladder was not ruptured, and her injury was isolated to a pelvic fracture. She was placed in traction and sent for CT imaging. Unfortunately, the CT revealed that the pelvis fracture was comminuted—or in too many pieces to simply place plates and screws to fix it. She needed an external fixator, commonly called a halo, which is basically an erector set used to hold multiple bone sources in place to allow for healing and stability.

On the way to the operating room, her next of kin showed up—a mid- to late 20s African American woman who wore her head shaved on both sides and floppy dreadlocks on the top. She seemed to be hardened from the streets, and because Samantha and her family all had concealed carry permits, she recognized the next of kin had a handgun in her beltline.

"Take care of my number one bitch," the next of kin yelled at the staff. "I've got to keep my track full." After unleashing some other expletives, she was escorted out by police, who told us that this was a unique situation; the next of kin was a well-known female pimp in our downtown area who ran young women from rural parts of our state to the city and put them in sleezy hotels and cars. She fed them drugs and made money off them when strangers paid to have sex with them. Samantha was in a haze from the sleep deprivation and didn't think anything of it.

At 3:30 a.m., Samantha went to the operating room with her attending, Dr. Puget. The case went as planned, and after a couple hours, they had pieced together as much of the pelvis as possible and attached the circular external fixator to pelvic bones with rings around her entire waste holding her pelvis and hips aligned and secured to keep the fragments from shifting. The procedure was uneventful, and Samantha put orders in to admit the patient to a room.

That morning on rounds the patient told Samantha (who was about to check out and go home since her shift was done) that she planned to leave that day. It's rare in our facility for an external fixator patient to leave the day after surgery, regardless of the location of the device, as pain is likely to increase and they need to be under observation.

Later that morning the next of kin showed up and yelled at the nurse, and the patient signed a form to leave AMA (against medical advice). She reported she would see Dr. Puget in the office for follow-up. External fixators typically come off after eight to twelve weeks; in this scenario, it would require a return trip to the operating room to remove the device.

Approximately six months later, Samantha was working the emergency department on call for house officer and was asked to admit a patient. The same young lady was back in the ER, this time with withdrawal from crack cocaine. The patient said her pelvis felt better, and she had just left the external fixator intact since she was last seen.

Samantha described the protocol that would follow to treat her withdrawal symptoms, saying that the patient would feel better in a couple days. The imaging of the pelvis showed that the fracture had healed—proof that young patients are made of rubber and can heal anything. The patient was already walking without assistance. Samantha said they would take her to the operating room to remove the external fixator, but the patient adamantly refused. Samantha asked why.

The young drug addict, prostitute, human-trafficking victim told Samantha business had never been better. She was put up in a hotel room and treated like royalty. The clients (or Johns) loved the external fixator on her pelvis, thinking of it as handlebars.

"I'm making over $2,000 a night fucking professional men, athletes, truck drivers, and before I was getting random $20 or $30 for blowjobs with broke men driving broken-down cars."

Samantha couldn't wrap her head around this. She told the patient she was concerned about human trafficking and was going to tell the hospital police. The patient begged her not to do that. Samantha went to the front police area, but by the time she walked back to the patient's room, she was gone, having left out the back of the emergency department.

She was never seen again and for all Samantha knows she still has the external fixator on if she didn't go to another hospital system for removal. Samantha's mind often drifts to this day and the marketing of prostitutes with handlebars, how some folks seemingly hit rock bottom and turn their life around while other people continue to spiral out of control. The fact that these folks walk amongst us is still a struggle for Samantha to understand.

CHAPTER 4
As Seen on TV

Although each of us interns went to different medical schools, we commonly were asked if being a medical student, resident, or physician was like *Grey's Anatomy*. This is a wildly popular television show about training physicians and surgeons at a hospital that mostly involves all of the doctors and healthcare workers having sex with each other and the drama that ensues.

Samantha was the most focused, efficient person you could hope to meet. There were no hours of the day that she didn't spend working, which was what led to her perfect scores on the MCAT (our admission test to medical school) and then on the in-training exam, an annual, national test all residents take to gauge learning progress. Samantha had been a college softball player, and David would say, "Based on the pantsuits you wear to meetings, I'm going to assume you're a lesbian." Whenever the nurses got breast reconstructions from one of the plastic surgeons, they inevitably invited Samantha into an empty patient room to inspect their new breasts. Samantha loved it, but she only looked scientifically at the repair and scar; there were never any sexual encounters.

David was a country boy with a wife of four years, three sons, plus a fourth on the way. He didn't have time or any desire to pursue an extramarital affair. He was clearly in love with his wife and family and worked hard at work, not wasting any time so he could get home sooner to his family.

Robert acted low key and reserved and would rather say he had only gotten this far with luck than hard work. However, Robert was not just a happy-go-lucky individual. To get into this program you have to be elite, and type A doesn't begin to describe these residents. Robert had the fewest book smarts and the most street smarts. He was a former Division 1 football player, and when asked about women, there was only one—and she had him wrapped around her finger.

Robert was captain of his college football team, class president, strong jawed and handsome, standing six feet eight and weighing 275 pounds of muscle. He had a smile that would light up the room. He had been ahead of his peers physically and with popularity his whole life. However, coming from a broken home where he lived in poverty, he never had the self-esteem his outward appearance portrayed. His co-residents would tell him, "Look! The nurses, staff, older female physicians, and cafeteria ladies that were anywhere from 18 to 70 years old are all throwing themselves at you." His drive came from his longtime girlfriend for whom he was head over heels, and he didn't even realize when others were flirting with him. Robert had been through the party scene in college in Miami, Florida, where he described sports parties, alcohol, and women, and even working for extra money in the off-season as a server at a Lifestyle Club. (For those that don't know that type of club, it's a members-only swingers club, and Robert essentially was being paid to have sex with married or lonely women and groups of women.)

His girlfriend was a year ahead of him in school, and although she was known as unattainable, they were getting married at the end of the intern year. She wasn't impressed with Robert, and that drove him to greatness. She was a tall blonde with crystal-blue eyes. She was in shape but supple, the kind of doctor that turns heads when she walks down the hallway, the one everyone stops and looks at in a meeting. Throughout the year, a couple of the attendings tried to get her to leave Robert, and these alpha males (who hadn't met Robert) tried to make her theirs. Although lacking self-esteem, Robert had grown up in the inner city and was a youth-league boxer who had turned to Brazilian jujitsu by his college years to work out his demons. The first time an attending cornered Robert's soon-to-be wife in a hallway of the hospital, she called Robert, crying. He immediately drove to the hospital. The residents aren't allowed in the physicians' lounge at our hospital, but Robert sweet-talked the nighttime security staff lady into letting him in.

After she opened the door, he quietly thanked her and smiled, and she was smitten and went back to her shift. Robert walked angrily to the attending physician—a slimy-looking, bug-eyed, chauvinist, loud-talking, arrogant surgeon at the hospital. The attending stood up when he saw a mountain of a man coming at him. The attending, standing all of five feet six inches and weighing 150 pounds wet, was shaken up. Robert grabbed the attending's white coat at the chest, pulled it together, and lifted this attending physician off the ground, pinning him against the wall. Robert told him in his gruff, deep voice that if he heard of him making a pass at his girlfriend and soon to be fiancée (or another student or resident female who was subservient to him), he would rip his small dick off and shove it down his throat. Believe it or not, the attending pissed himself and started crying. Robert put him back in the chair and stormed off.

The next day Robert was called to the medical education department to talk to administration. He was in trouble, but the attending's ego was too large to press charges; plus, the head of general surgery was sitting at the computer next to the attending when Robert walked in the night before. He was an old cowboy who wore his boots on rounds and had no idea this attending had been abusing his position of power with younger women for years. Robert was excused and told to never assault anyone again; if he did, he would be terminated from the residency program. He told the medical education director, "If I assaulted him, we'd be having this conversation at the prison or graveside." He explained he was just sending a message and could have killed the attending if he wanted to. The general surgeon launched an investigation against the attending, during which many victims came out during the MeToo movement. The attending was dismissed from the hospital.

The interns would talk about *Grey's Anatomy*, and the public thought they were all freaks. However, as anyone who works in a hospital will tell you, the freaks are the nurses and security guards. There was a whole group of male security guards and young nurses who were sleeping with each other throughout the hospital.

We would walk by empty patient rooms and hear moaning and grunting from the room, look at each other, shake our heads, and say, "Yeah, *Grey's Anatomy* over there doesn't remember the last patient in there died and had MRSA and C. diff. That's some dirty sex right there!"

When we had our resident didactics or learning, such as journal clubs, meeting with radiology, or other residency activities, and they started in the education conference room earlier than the scheduled 4:00 p.m. time, we would walk into our conference room and see one of the security guards with a nurse.

This security guard was a ripped former cop who had gotten in trouble during some vice work on prostitution. Women, including nurses, love a man in uniform, and nurses also want to help someone. He played the broken-man card and was in impeccable physical shape, and he went through nurses like you wouldn't believe. Tim (the guard) would admit he was dumb as a brick, but he was hung like a horse and was an adventurist. Apparently, many of the nurses were adventurists too. Every Wednesday we would get there early just to see. We would key into the conference room with our ID badges, and there was Tim, his security belt down past his waist, a nurse with her scrubs off sitting on the filing cabinet or table with Tim nailing her.

There they were, always in a wet, steamy session, and Tim would say, "My bad again, guys." He and the nurse would get dressed and scurry out, Tim always thanking us as he left. We wondered where they would go next to continue—maybe the morgue! The problem was there was always a different nurse, so during our intern year, we counted he was with at least 50 different nurses or staff women. Since we weren't anywhere near living the Grey's Anatomy life, we affectionately referred to our security guard friend as McTimmy!

CHAPTER 5
Checkered Past

David was on the general surgery service and got a call on a patient with a large leg abscess. Part of taking house officer rotations includes educating medical students who are ending their education with hospital rounds after doing intense classwork. They are the nervous people wearing short white coats stuffed with items, who are wondering who is going to "pimp" them next. ("Pimping," as it is termed, is when residents, fellows, and attending (established doctors) ask questions in a grilling fashion. Picture academic boot camp with a stress for perfection. A lot can be learned in this heightened sense.)

We refer to this as "education by humiliation." If you're embarrassed, you'll remember. Ever had a traumatic event in your life? I bet you remember all the details, even though you try push it to the back of your mind. Well, this works great with education as well.

The student was a beautiful woman named Emily, currently in her last year at the local state medical school. As a Level 1 trauma center, students from throughout the country rotate through. She was a former college varsity cheerleader and a true knockout. Smart and sexy, she was appealing to most of the male doctors and staff, yet still vulnerable. She was nervous and wanted to do a good job, thinking our hospital was where she may want to be an intern then a resident in general surgery.

Unfortunately, Emily had a bad habit of thinking she was farther along in her training than she was. She would skip steps and try to rush to prove her abilities. (This is dangerous if someone is trying to take care of your family member.) David knew this, and in his southern twang, he said her abilities were "big hat, no cattle" (southern for all show and no backing).

David was assigned to teach students on morning rounds. As medical students, they are in their third or fourth year of medical school, having made it through the classroom work and boards to where the real learning starts in the hospital. However, David was still learning too, and sometimes medical students can be more of a hassle than an asset and put you in a tough situation.

Emily was a gunner, a student shooting to be number one at all costs, on the rotation with David. The student was given three patients to look up, chart, prepare, and see with David, the remainder of the 15 patients on David's service for which he was in charge. David and the student pre-rounded on the patient and prepared for the arrival of the attending (the doctor in charge of patients and whose name was assigned to those patients) for official rounds. (This is why when you're in the hospital so many people come in your room early in the morning; it's part of teaching.)

The gunner student went to an elite New England college and medical school, the kind of person who spent her whole life in and around the one percent population. She always reminded us that her father was the CEO of a Fortune 500 company and her mother was a general surgeon in Massachusetts. The student would always say that her parents' careers made her middle class in the neighborhood where she grew up. The student was unbeknownst to her living a sociology experiment, thrusting her elite background and socioeconomic level into our inner-city, dirty hospital! I don't think she was ever told no or that she was wrong. She walked with grace and arrogance.

David was the exact opposite of this student, and they butted heads often. She reviewed her patients in a hurry and had this "I got everything under control" look on her face. Off they went to see the first patient. Little did she know David had studied the patient too and picked up a subtle but important past-medical-history finding that he didn't think she caught. He wanted to keep a close eye on the student.

The student, Emily, hadn't read the patient's past medical history before going in to see the 57-year-old male. He had been living at a homeless shelter and had bites all along his lower legs bilaterally. Suspicion was for bedbugs with superimposed staph infection cellulitis. Emily, the former cheerleader and arrogant student, pulled the ends of the sheets up, put on gloves, and started examining the patient's legs. For suspected bedbug bites, we have to wear protective gowns, hats, gloves, and shoes to prevent spread. The room was sanitized.

As Emily started examining the patient's legs, David noticed the sheets were going up and down at the patient's midsection. David chuckled and smiled.

Emily looked up at him, saying, "What's wrong with you today?!"

"Oh nothing," David said, "just thinking through this patient's medical history and your care."

The sheets were moving more violently, and the patient started to actually laugh and giggle. Emily shrugged him off and started to describe her findings. "This is a maculopapular rash with resolving cellulitis. No full wounds or obvious bites." She paused. "Oh my God, HELP!" She threw off her gloves and all the protective gear and ran out of the room and down the hall.

David went after her. She went into the patient family bathroom, and he could hear her vomiting and crying.

Jokingly, David said, "Emily, did you find a bedbug?!"

Emily said no through the bathroom door and asked David to leave.

David knew sanitation had removed the bedbugs. He also knew what was in the patient's medical history. "Hey, Emily, I bet you don't rush reading through the patient's chart thinking you know it all next time. This could have been avoided. I can't believe you didn't read his history of chronic public masturbation."

When Emily looked up from examining the patient's legs, right before she rushed from the room, she saw this man staring down at her and masturbating into the sheets. We joke as a class that she probably reads the past medical history at least three times now before she walks into a patient's room. Education and humility come in all forms.

CHAPTER 6
Teamwork Makes the Dream Work

Today, patients want to record their encounters with doctors for various reasons, including but not limited to filing lawsuits, streaming the encounter live on social media, and documenting pictures before and after. Patients who record procedures in the operating room, endoscopy procedures, dental sedations, and others are well within their rights; however, the acceptability of it is up for debate. Many things said in the operating room can be taken out of context.

Robert was scheduled to work with an established, renowned heart surgeon who not only published articles and textbooks but also ran a training program for elite general surgery residents selected for the fellowship in cardiothoracic surgery. The program was for the kind of high-octane, smart, driven people who want to crack open chests in emergency situations as well as during scheduled surgeries. Simply put, these doctors typically have nerves of steel. Sometimes surgeons become more popular thanks to their academic side, through writing and publishing, though they are not as skilled in practice. Many times, you would prefer to have the practitioner who does the most cases instead of the practitioner who has the time to publish the most articles.

Robert heard the cardiothoracic surgeon was cool, calm, and professional with patients, which contrasted with who he was in the operating room—a high-strung, nervous wreck when it came time to perform surgeries. Many times in the operating room, particularly with ill patients and given the tort lawsuit, medical malpractice driven society in which we live, you can cut the tension with a knife. The attendings use humor to break up this tension and calm themselves. Well, the attending Robert worked with was one of the best cardiothoracic surgeons in the world—of all time—and couldn't lower himself to tomfoolery and jokes.

Other attendings with whom Robert worked would joke throughout cases and discuss current events, operating under the laughter-is-the-best-medicine policy. There were even others that were like a fraternity, hitting on the nursing staff and scrub techs, blaring AC/DC, and running around having fun. Yet there was a small subset who listened to classical or jazz music and had complete focus, noted with silence in the OR, and even used hand signals to ask for different tools so that no one had to talk. (This also enables deaf people to work as scrub techs as they only need hand signals and is somewhat common in many hospitals.)

Rooms are stacked next to each other in the operating room suites with what's called a "sub-sterile"—a small room that doesn't require complete sterility, say between operating room 1 and operating room 2. You wear a cap in a sub-sterile, but you don't need a mask or gown. Typically, this is where towels, blankets, personal protective equipment, sharps containers, sinks, and autoclaves (to sterilize instruments) are kept. Picture a small, 10-foot-by-5-foot room with this equipment and two windowless doors that swing open and shut.

On his first week on the rotation, Robert had worked up a 62-year-old diabetic smoker with known peripheral vascular disease. The patient needed a four-vessel graft, a coronary artery bypass graft (or a CABG), commonly referred to as a bypass. The patient had been airlifted to the hospital from an outlying hospital two hours away for this emergent surgery required to keep the patient alive. It was roughly 2:00 p.m., and the patient had been signed by the attending "world's greatest" heart surgeon, and consent was completed.

There stood Robert in the operating room, waiting on this surgeon whose pager and cell phone were on the shelf, which meant he wasn't answering. Robert was getting nervous. Anesthesia was being introduced, and they were shaving and prepping the patient. The vitals were unstable, and the perfusionist and anesthesia team were keeping the patient stable until surgery could begin. The patient's extremities were starving for oxygenated blood given the lack of perfusion. Robert continued to wait, unable to hear a thing as his heart was pounding in his ears.

He turned to the scrub tech and knew he must have been white as a ghost, thinking he may have to break all the rules and start this surgery himself, a farfetched idea since he hadn't studied the anatomy on a cadaver in four years and didn't do well in cardiology classes.

The scrub tech chuckled at Robert and said, "What's your problem? You know Nurse Molly is getting the attending ready. Calm down and go scrub."

Robert went to the scrub sink and was using a scrub brush to clean out any debris under his nails, finishing off with a chemical (chlorhexidine) to kill off any bacteria. Sleep-deprived, Robert was drifting mentally, pondering that they scrubbed their hands with this disinfectant and wore gloves and gowns for sterile technique, but they were still washing their hands in city water. He thought there had to be a better way.

As he went on daydreaming, the attending appeared—all smiles—and slapped him on the back. "Let's do this, Robert," he said. The attending was ecstatic and all over the place mentally; he was in a great mood. "Hot lights, cold steel!" he continued. "Let's heal with steel! And remember, Robert, all bleeding eventually stops! Let's go help this guy. He'll let his friends know, and they'll want help too." It was a word salad of surgeon jargon.

The attending flew into the room, and Robert followed. The case went incredibly smoothly. The anesthesia team was caring for the patient and doing live echo through the esophagus. Everyone was in a good mood, including the perfusionist, scrub tech, first assistant, and the circulating nurse, Molly, who was in her late 20s and about five feet tall. She was tight-bodied former gymnast who had obviously had breast implants, and her red hair flowed out of her surgery bonnet cap.

The case was done, and the patient successfully went to recovery and eventually to the intensive care unit until he was ready for a normal floor. Robert went into the staff lounge where they ate lunch, chasing the scrub tech.

"What are you doing, coming in here with us?" the tech asked him.

Robert explained he just had to know what she meant when she said, "Molly was getting the surgeon ready." The attending was a nervous wreck prior to surgery, and then everything went perfect. Robert had heard of attending surgeons taking performance drugs, such as those given to narcoleptics, to focus and stay sharp mentally. He had even seen them take medications intended for ADHD, but he didn't know what could have been done to calm the surgeon. No one would take anti-anxiety pills before surgery; that would lead to the surgeon not remembering what happened and being too fatigued. Robert was sure there was no alcohol in the sub-sterile.

The scrub tech explained to Robert that the attending cardiothoracic surgeon started to develop problems with nerves, which was normal for any heart surgeon. Everyone knows going into it that many patients will still die, even if you do your best. The surgeon had real trouble dealing with this and with the family members of the patients that expired.

The scrub tech said, "It all started when Molly got that ridiculous boob job! After her breast surgery, the attending was joking one day before a surgery case, saying, 'Let's go in the sub-sterile and let me see those new tits!' Well, that's exactly what Molly did.

"So, we have a young, prominent, high-powered heart surgeon and a young, voluptuous nurse," the tech continued. "What do you think started to happen?" The scrub tech paused and then said, "Mostly I hear it's blow jobs before surgery."

Robert was shocked at how matter-of-fact she was about this. Robert knew the surgeon had been married since he was 18 years old and was a self-described Sunday-school-attending Christian. Molly also had a young son.

The scrub tech said, "You know Molly's son is the surgeon's, right?"

As it turned out, the surgeon's wife knew her husband had fathered Molly's child, and somehow they made this work. The attending surgeon and his wife, who had two children of their own, paid for Molly's son care, her mortgage, and other bills. Apparently, what was initially kept quiet had eventually gotten out, as Molly bragged to other staff about how she was taken care of financially. Robert couldn't wrap his head around this.

The scrub tech said, "Believe it because it's true, and that's not the worst scandal we've had around here. Before your time, Robert, there was a female surgery resident who got pregnant. There were three attendings who were all in the same general surgery practice together, and she didn't know which one was the father. Worse yet, the surgeons didn't know she was having sex with all of them. They were oblivious. It turns out if you're a nympho working in a hospital with type A, competitive, wealthy, hot surgeons like yourself, Robert, it's a feeding frenzy!"

The scrub tech also told Robert about a plastic surgeon who was in his 70s at their hospital who was on his sixth wife; they had an eight-year-old son together. The surgeon had married nurses and slept with numerous other ones at the same hospital, essentially trading them in as the women got older. He was struggling financially because of this, which was why he was working so hard at his age (he had numerous children and ex-wives). Unfortunately, his sixth wife had just filed for divorce. Apparently, he was caught in a Craigslist sex encounter with a couple of hookers and a large amount of cocaine.

Robert shook his head, thinking, *Doctors aren't immune to the human fault, and maybe they are more prone to it because of the stress. After all, suicide rates for physicians and surgeons have gone through the roof recently.*

Robert said out loud, "Oh well, I'm in too deep with my student loans to stop now, and I don't have any other skill set. See you tomorrow!"

CHAPTER 7
Roll the Dice

Sex injuries are common, and in the emergency department they are often labeled as "ear infection," a label that holds until the doctor arrives; then it becomes an STD or an injury while having sex. The patient doesn't want to tell anyone but the doctor the real reason for the visit. The most common at this hospital were testicular torsion and broken penis; however, even worse sexual injuries can occur.

Within walking distance to the hospital, a new casino was built, and initially, the hospital held meetings for physicians, staff, and residents/interns in their meeting space. However, this quickly stopped as hospital staff on the way in and out were subjected to many frequent-flyer patients (people who come in all the time). Not only was this a nuisance, but it was also a security risk, so the hospital stopped using the meeting space.

David was on the general surgery house officer rotation and covering for colorectal for the weekend. Right before dinner on a Friday night, the first patient from the casino and adjoining hotel came in. She was 34 years old and slightly overweight, and she was wearing a dress and heels and glitter makeup. She had been at the casino and hotel since the night prior. She was having pain that she hadn't experienced before and was septic. It turned out she had an infection and gangrene.

She had necrotizing fasciitis of her perineum. (The perineum is the anatomical structure between your anus and your genitals in both males and females.) This condition is typically caused by bacteria that don't need oxygen to survive, and it can lead to significant amputation; it can be deadly, even in healthy patients. The common name for the condition is "flesh-eating bacteria." In other words, bacteria were eating through her layers of skin, fat, muscle, and eventually the pelvis and all structures between her vagina and anus. Because this infection eventually works itself into the rectum and colon, not only is there pus, there is also feces, which can lead to an ungodly smell that hits you 30 feet before you walk into the room.

The patient had risk factors and was deteriorating. Any delay in care would lead to permanent dysfunction, chronic pain, and death, so David rushed to surgery with the colorectal team. The patient was debrided, and plans for a wound vac (a device that allows healing from the inside out with suction) and transfer to the floor were established. As he finished writing the orders, it was after midnight, and he was paged from the emergency department. Annoyed more than anything else, he returned the call.

"What's the consult for?" he asked.

"Fornier's gangrene perineum, 28-year-old female," was the reply.

David thought this was strange, so he headed right down. This patient had a very similar presentation with newer onset necrotizing fasciitis, and of course, it was at her perineum. He called the attending colorectal surgeon and told him not to go home, then he prepared the patient and went to surgery for debridement. This patient would go on to have a long hospital course with multiple surgeries, requiring a specialist to reconstruct her anus and genitalia. She was asked how this occurred, and the patient reported she was partying with friends at the casino. *That doesn't make sense*, David thought.

After this surgery David looked on the board and saw three perineum abscesses pending admit through the emergency department. He fielded all the calls at once and said, "You've got to be kidding me." Of course these types of infections can spread rapidly, as surgeons like to say "time is tissue!" The infection can be mild at first and less than an hour later be life threatening so treatment is expedited and not delayed.

He went into the emergency department, and the stench was unbelievable. He applied Mastisol, a chemical used as an adherent, to a surgical mask so that the chemical was all he could smell. It was 3:30 a.m., and all the women were in their mid- to late 20s; they were done up for going out; however, they were in pain, febrile, and they were all septic and needed surgery immediately. David called the attending, who brought one of his partners in for the cases, as well as a fellow in colorectal training and another resident. They opened up two operating rooms to accommodate. The difficult decision as to who to take first was based not on their arrival but on how stable they were.

Before completing consent forms and heading to surgery, David stopped and said, "Wait a minute." He went into each room and asked the patients how this happened. Each said they had been partying at the casino with friends and staying at the hotel. Finally, the last patient said she met a smooth, Hispanic guy named Hector and they hit it off at the bar. The next thing she knew, she agreed to go to his hotel room and had sex with him. He was in his 40s and promised her the world.

39

He told the physician assistant, "Is the fucking these ladies are getting worth the fucking they're going to get? There's some rotting dick over at the casino!" Then David went back to each room and asked, "Was there a guy named Hector?" Indeed, over the past three days, they had all had sex with Hector.

David told the story to Robert who was taking over the list in the early morning, and he was in disbelief, thinking David must have been overworked and was making this up. Five patients in one night with perineum gangrene and all because of one man?

Robert finished morning rounds, and the patients were stable. He was then paged to the emergency department, and the consult was for "bad penis." Robert didn't think anything of it until he looked at the chart before walking in the room: Hector Martinez. *You have got to be kidding me*, Robert thought. Hector was a 40-something Hispanic who was here in the U.S. on a work visa and living with family.

Not only did Hector test positive for syphilis, herpes, genital warts, and chlamydia, he also had a raging fungal infection in his groin commonly seen in developing countries. This explained the unprotected sex and the numerous women coming into the emergency department.

Hector had a long stay in the hospital, which cleared his penis and genitals, and he eventually was deported to Mexico. David and Robert never saw the female patients again, but to this day they refer to the casino as Hector's Poker Place!

CHAPTER 8
Young Love

A 17-year-old male patient was admitted for opioid withdrawal and started on the protocol to wean him from the drug. His girlfriend, who was 16, moved into the room with him. Both were homeless, neither had bathed in quite some time, and both were heroin addicts.

The opioid-addiction crisis is an epidemic plaguing not just inner cities but spreading throughout the country and even into farming and rural areas. The classic scenario we see in the hospital is addicts coming in to get away from the streets or because they're in withdrawal. All too often, the younger partner, the girl in this case, falls in love with the older partner, and they start using. Money gets short, and he starts selling her on the streets. She turns tricks for cash so they can both get high.

When asked why he used heroin, the boy said because it "takes you to the moon." He was a popular kid—a football star and homecoming king. He said he wasn't afraid of anything, including heroin. The first time he tried it, it was enough to hook him for life. Now this young girl was staying in the bed with him or sleeping in a bedside chair.

Patients lust for opioids, and we have to get past that thirst for the drug in the hospital while safely protecting them from withdrawal, which can kill them itself. Because the relapse rate among heroin users is significant, we call our treatment of them something more akin to remission than recovery; they tend to relapse and chase that high again.

This patient said he always had to have his next fix, meaning while he was high, he had to score more heroin—say, before going to bed—so that when he woke up, his next fix was right there on the nightstand.

The patient had now been almost 24 hours without opioids and was withdrawing and in misery—sweating, hurting, hallucinating, and begging for opioids. His young lover saw an opportunity. She knew that patients in the hospital often pretend to take their pain pills and then sell them in the hospital, so she started asking around.

Many times, diabetics with neuropathy come in with foot infections and fractures that they can't feel. However, they say they're in pain so that they can get the oral pain medications, and then they sell them. This young woman purchased oxycodone-acetaminophen from one of these diabetic patients. She wanted to help her beloved boyfriend as quickly as possible.

The 16-year-old girl decided that if her boyfriend swallowed the pills, they would have little effect because his high required extreme, daily doses of heroin. She also thought snorting it would be impossible because he was combative in withdrawal. So, what did she do? She ground up the pills and grabbed a saline syringe from the room. (Heroin addicts know the supplies and how to find veins. We say they would be great phlebotomists, and some phlebotomists—those who draw blood—are former addicts.) This time, though, she didn't need to find a vein. She had a main access to his IV.

She injected the ground-up heroin into her boyfriend's peripheral IV, and his EKG monitor started to alert and alarm. She started crying and yelling for help. The patient was turning blue, and the floor nurse called a code.

A code stands for any urgent matter, and there are numerous types. Code blue is the most dreaded as it means the person is actively dying; sometimes you can help, and sometimes you can't. There is nothing worse than a code pager going off. If you've ever felt your fight-or-flight response kick in, say in a schoolyard tussle, exponentially increase that. When you hear the sound of that pager, your mind starts racing, and when you get there, you have tunnel vision. Your training kicks in, and everything becomes instinctual because you've practiced it over and over. You can't think, so you go into autopilot. Then you notice the family at the patient's bedside, and in this case it's a young, drug-addicted, beautiful young woman with a lost soul.

The code team consists of nurses, respiratory techs, anesthesia, physicians, and ancillary staff with folks documenting and timing. Samantha is on the code team and is running to the scene, literally going through the differentials the patient could have and what could be done. The differentials didn't add up, so Samantha asked the girl what happened. She said she didn't know.

They started giving epinephrine and chest compressions. They put on the AED, drew blood, and went into heroic-measures mode. With the stat imaging they determined that perhaps there was a clot and administered thrombolytics, which are meant to bust apart a clot. (We have developed ways to break apart cholesterol clots using pharmaceuticals, but we don't have any way to break apart a piece of oxycodone.)

The girlfriend screamed and yelled for the team to help her young lover. She begged them, falling to her knees and admitting what she'd done. Samantha and her team stopped the code and watched the 17-year-old boy die. It was the hardest thing she'd ever experienced, watching a young, healthy life die in front of her, knowing there was nothing she could do to stop it. The injection of those pieces of the drug went into the larger arteries just fine as debris. However, once they got to smaller arteries in all the organs—including the heart and the brain—they blocked the blood flow. He died quickly.

The other part of a code being run is security, and these officers usually keep the peace during a high-stress time. They were on the scene for this code, and right or wrong (you be the judge), the 16-year-old girl was taken into custody to be charged with murder. Samantha felt like two lives were lost that night, one to death and one to dependence. Perhaps the girl will get the help she needs, serve her time, and make a life for herself, looking back at this as a bad dream.

Samantha intermittently followed the young girl's progress in the courts during our intern year. She was tried as an adult, though she was granted some leniency because of the situation and no proof of intent; his family decided not to press charges and give her a chance. Unexpectedly, she showed back up at our OB/GYN unit nine months later, sober and still in custody, and delivered her and her deceased boyfriend's daughter. The baby wasn't on heroin protocol and was going to be raised by her grandparents. With death comes life, a life this 17-year-old boy never knew about.

CHAPTER 9
Bathing in Bath Salts

Somehow many of our inner-city patients were slow to get the memo about bath salts being bad for them. Apparently, someone was pushing these drugs on the streets near the hospital, and when David went on house officer nights, they were inundated with these patients.

It was common to see patients naked and with scratches all over their bodies from running through the woods. One of these was a door-to-door salesman who liked bath salts and Four Lokos because he could do his shift quicker with these speed balls. David could only imagine a drugged-up, sweating, running, fast-talking salesman.

"You know, where I come from," David said to the patient, "we shoot people like you who knock on our door uninvited."

The patients typically were like zombies, writhing around, both their hands and feet tied, their back arching as they tried to free themselves from the bed. With their heart racing, all we could do was monitor them and wait for the high to pass. They all came down hard from the high and went into a deep sleep, waking up to sadness and amnesia regarding what had occurred.

Each operating room is equipped with cameras and microphones that feed into monitors in the surgeons' lounge. You can click on these, and the operating room you choose takes over the whole screen; you can see and hear what's occurring. David really enjoyed this, especially on weekend nights. He would turn on the evening news and watch both the news and the operating room, feeling that he knew something society didn't; he was ahead of the public information.

David was watching when a beautiful, well-kept female news anchor came on, and with a sparkle in her eye and wearing a happy, perfect smile said, "A young man was shot during a robbery attempt gone wrong. The man is said to be in critical condition but alive."

Alone in the surgeons' lounge, David yelled out, "No! He's dead!" He had been watching the operating room surgeon and staff working in real time on the patient the news anchor was describing. He had seen them in Operating Room 3 exhaust their efforts and throw in the towel, pronouncing the patient dead. No one except for the medical staff and physicians were aware the patient had died. He would not go through a trial, he wouldn't serve any jail time. There would be no closure, no last words.

David stood up, and his pager went off. The ICU staff needed the house officer to evaluate a patient. It was about bath salts. He grappled with the thought of the 18-year-old who just died in the operating room and another life wasting away from likely drug addiction.

When he arrived in the ICU, he saw an overweight, dirty, 50-something-year-old woman tweaking on the ICU bed. She was in restraints and being held down by security staff and patient assistants. And they had brought in a cage, which stopped David in his tracks. He had never seen a person put in a cage before.

The cage is a soft shelter enclosing a bed that is approximately six-by-six-by-five feet. It is secured on all sides, and there is netting or mesh at the front. There is a small zipper the size of a basketball at the front that can be opened to reach patients, and open sleeves in the mesh enable the examination of patients.

Security and staff transferred the patient and tied her into what is essentially a prison cell, though it was done for her own good. In the process of transferring her, she kicked a staff member in the face and bit a security guard. She was high on bath salts and had unbelievable strength, though she was sweating and exhausted.

David tried to speak with the patient, but she just spit on him and hissed. Before the restraints were applied, she had been throwing feces at the staff, which is an all-too-common occurrence in the psychiatric ward or when patients are on drugs. He asked the nurse and intensivist (the ICU doctor) for an update.

The patient, a crack cocaine addict, had been renting a space via Airbnb, living in someone's garage. After a crack cocaine binge, her dealer offered her bath salts. Apparently, she liked getting high (like a heroin addict) to near death, when Narcan is used to resuscitate these addicts. (Makes me wonder if Europe's program of providing clean needles and treating addiction as a mental illness is the correct model of care.)

Many times, the Reagan administration is mentioned around the hospital and blamed for closing insane asylums, which resulted in these schizophrenics and patients with other psychiatric disorders walking the streets. The patients don't feel safe, and neither does society. This patient was likely one of these people. You don't end up in a garage using crack cocaine and bath salts without at least a mental breakdown and more likely a mental illness. The nurse reported the patient had been like this for two days and wasn't getting any better.

The owner of the house who had leased her the space in their garage heard some strange noises in the garage and then a thud. When they entered the garage, the patient was unresponsive on the cement floor. There was a hole in the drywall and drywall debris in her mouth; she had been eating her way out. They called 911 and the patient went into rhabdomyolysis, which is when muscles waste away when the patient is down for too long, which leads to renal failure.

"You've got to be kidding me," David said. "This lady is nuttier than squirrel shit!"

So she was high on bath salts—yes, the same drug that reportedly caused someone to eat another person's face in Miami, Florida—and she couldn't get the drug out of her system because her kidneys weren't working. She was on a never-ending high because her body couldn't get rid of the bath-salt toxins.

These are new drugs, there is no literature out on how to treat someone in this condition, so David called the nephrologist (the kidney specialist) who was on call. These doctors provide rounding services and are rarely called into the hospital in the middle of the night, particularly on weekends. The on-call nephrologist was a former college and pro football player and was considered a gentle giant. However, he was also an evangelical Christian who was known to struggle with patients whose life views differed from his. Regardless of all that, David called and talked to the nephrologist, pleading his case for urgent dialysis to try to get the kidneys functioning so that they could clear the bath salts from this patient's system.

The nephrologist told David he wasn't missing sleep over a patient who had done this to herself. It was a routine consult, and he had 24 hours to see the patient. He was right that it likely wasn't going to make a difference in the patient's outcome. All her organs were at risk at this point, regardless of treatment.

David hung up the phone and put his head on the desk. He knew the rest of the night he was going to babysit this patient and try to keep her alive until the kidney specialist saw her in the morning and started dialysis.

So, David embarked on the night that his fellow interns would later call "David's night of the living dead." He spent the entire night with a human being who was at their most primitive core, unable to perform higher-level thinking, truly a living zombie on earth. Human resilience, the patient survived although she ended up dependent on dialysis lifelong. Now likely having a more painful and depressing life than before, this made David think did he really do the patient a favor by keeping her alive that night.

CHAPTER 10
Not a Flash Mob

The hospital system that we were in unfortunately had not connected all electronic medical records, and there were multiple other hospital systems in our city. This meant that with this antiquated communication, if a patient came from another hospital only five miles away, we would have to request records and often wait up to five business days to get the record. In the business world five days may not seem like a long time, but in healthcare it's high risk and an eternity.

Imagine a patient walks into the emergency department and your hospital has no records for them. They have an obvious scar and are having complications. You try to call the hospital where they were previously treated and get no response. Who knows if the patient is even telling you the right hospital? You have to treat this patient blindly until records arrive.

In many hospitals, especially outlying smaller facilities, this is still commonplace. Only this year did our system get the ability to share electronic records throughout the system and see other hospitals' information on the patient (even though this might be limited). Hopefully the correct Social Security information and name were given, and if that was the case, the outside records (as we refer to records not in the system) could be found. Around our hospital it was common to hear doctors saying, "What did the outside internist [or the outside surgeon] do for this patient?" This is especially prevalent at a Level 1 trauma center like ours as outside doctors and specialists tend to dump patients on the larger hospital for the weekends.

Consider this scenario: A patient with appendicitis comes into a rural hospital on a late Friday night. The general surgeon at the rural hospital (who isn't used to coming to the hospital in middle of night) says this patient is too complex or risky. They ask that the patient be sent to the tertiary hospital, such as ours. The patient then arrives in distress and with no documentation after a couple hours in an ambulance. The imaging typically has to be redone, and assumptions are made and care started. If they are able to advocate for themselves at all, patients should always get paperwork from the first hospital when being transferred.

Samantha was on house officer when a nurse called her to a room. When she appeared, every security guard and policeman in the hospital was outside the room. She briefly checked the patient chart and saw that he was being worked up for metastatic cancer. When Samantha pushed through the staff, she walked into the room and saw a "cancer patient." (It's hard to describe, but when you see a patient fighting metastatic disease, you know it immediately. They're emaciated, their tissues are wasting, their skin is sunken on their bones, their eyes are withdrawn and darkening, their skin is dehydrated, and they're frail and weak, to name a few descriptors.) The patient was a 48-year-old man who appeared to be on the mountaintop, near death.

Next to the patient sat an Italian man in his 50s in a three-piece suit, and two things struck Samantha about this visitor: one was the size of the diamond on his pinky ring and the other was the clearly visible handgun and holster under his suit jacket. He had a smile on his face and introduced himself politely to Samantha as the patient's guardian and even kissed her on the cheek, which she did not expect. The issue was that a tech had caught the patient hiding his pain medication after being given it to take. Apparently, he put it under his tongue, drank the water, and then tucked it in the filing cabinet next to the bed. The Italian gentlemen was discussing this with the cops and security guards, asking them to let this slide as he was "clearly saving it for the nighttime when he had the most pain."

The patient was warned, and Samantha continued his cancer work-up, involving the oncologist and surgeon, and planning for staged procedure and imaging. Later in the house officer shift, the hospital sent an email announcement reporting the hospital could now connect to other hospital systems for patient records. Samantha decided to see what the patient's diagnosis was, as he clearly had cancer.

She scrolled through lists of the same imaging being done over and over and progress notes from at least eight hospitals nearby showing the same cancer work-up; the patient reported he had been told the cancer had metastasized at the last hospital. A large portion of oral opioids had been given to this patient as his narcotic score was at the top of the screen. This didn't faze Samantha; cancer patients are routinely in significant pain and require large doses of opioids. The patient had requested pills, saying they worked better than IV pain medication, which usually signified he wasn't an abuser who was looking for the rush of IV pain medication. At our hospital, we had a policy for nurses to slowly deliver IV opioids (including Dilaudid and morphine), and daily we saw patients ask them to push it faster as they were chasing the high.

Samantha thought something wasn't right about this patient, and then she found the note—a single note buried amongst many by a behavioral health physician, which is what we now call psychiatrists. The psychiatrist had met with the patient one-on-one, much to his caretaker's disagreement. The patient admitted to the psychiatrist that he had gotten involved with the Mafia.

Because he looked like a cancer patient, his job was to travel the United States and go to all the hospitals in one area before moving to their next city. He would pretend to be a cancer patient until either the records came in from another hospital or his work-up showed no cancer. He was perfectly healthy and just looked severely ill, which the Mafia had capitalized on. All day he would get high-dosed oral opioids, stash them away, and give them to the mobster who was labeled as his caretaker. These were then put on the street for sale. This patient and the mob operation were responsible for a significant amount of oral opioids being on the street in any area they worked.

Being strong-willed and known for not being afraid of anything, Samantha went storming into the room. "You have some nerve pretending to be a cancer patient," she said. "You have no ethics or morals and you're being discharged."

The patient and the mobster were polite and thanked her for letting them know. They collected their belongings—which she was certain included a day's worth of high-dosed oral opioids—packed up and walked out, the patient leaving in the hospital gown.

Samantha shook her head as she watched them walk past security and onto the elevator. She couldn't imagine in today's society that this could be your role, that you could be so down on your luck you fall prey to this con. Then she thought there was no way to red flag the chart, and unless someone happened to stumble on this psychiatrist's note, they'd likely never know.

This is a con that will continue to travel the country. Don't believe everything you hear and only half of what you see. Samantha feared retaliation from the Mafia for messing up their supply line, to which David said, "Don't worry about it. They're likely in another state by now working this con."

CHAPTER 11
Miranda Who?

David was on the house officer rotation and rounding on a cold winter weekend morning. Snow was falling, and the wind was howling. Expecting a lot of head trauma and slip-and-fall injuries, he went to see a patient admitted for chest pain. The troponins, which are labs to evaluate the heart, were not elevated, and the patient had normal diagnostic results. However, the patient's drug toxicology screen was positive for cocaine. The patient, a Hispanic male in his late 40s who reported living in the city with his cousins, had moved here from Mexico. He reported being afraid to be in the hospital, thinking this put him at risk for deportation, and he discussed with David the United States building a wall.

David told him that he would be in observation for the remainder of the day and then likely discharged to head home. As David walked out of the patient's room, he saw a small scale by the window and thought that was odd. Because the patient was mildly obese and a type 2 diabetic, the good-hearted intern thought that perhaps he was weighing his food for a diet.

As he was walking down the hall, David was paged to the emergency department. *Another drug-problem patient*, he thought.

David spoke with the emergency department physician, who reported it was a 21-year-old male with a terrible infection in his penis. David quickly asked why he was called and not urology. The answer surprised naïve David, who matured a lot during this day in residency. The patient had injected his penis with heroin. When the patient was asked why he would inject his penis, he responded that he had nowhere else to do it.

Many of the patients David had seen during his intern year were "skin poppers," meaning they didn't access veins for heroin use; they simply injected their skin wherever they wanted. This patient, however, was precise and chased a stronger high by injecting directly in his veins. Many times, patients come into the hospital to get an IV line—or worse, a central line—and then leave against medical advice. They don't tell anyone they're leaving. One minute they're heading outside to smoke, and the next minute they're gone. This is dangerous because they have direct access to shoot up heroin.

David knew the heroin epidemic was bad throughout the country. He had read a book and some news articles that described how Mexican cartels had identified cities with dwindling cocaine sales where an opioid crisis was occurring due to prescription pain pills and that the cartels had put Mexicans in these places to sell heroin.

This patient was a nice-looking rural kid who was in shape and came from a good family. He was a football player and on the board for his 4-H group in high school. A young woman was with the patient at his bedside; she looked to be a similar age, although her disheveled appearance and sunken eyes made her appear older. She had obviously been living a rough life. Fittingly she was the high school cheerleading captain during the patient's senior year, and they had been dating for three years. She covered the scars on her arms well, but she was obviously hooked on heroin as well.

The patient reported an all-too-common history of taking small doses of pain pills, which escalated to craving larger doses of opioids. The patient had an ACL tear his junior year of high school and underwent a repair with one of our nation's leading orthopedists. He was given the common protocol of a short course of post-operative pain medication. The problem with the "sixth vital sign" (as pain is called) is there is no way to objectively measure the patient's pain level. It's not all big pharmaceutical companies that are driving doctor's decisions; it's a patient in pain in front of you and your compassion and oath to help them.

Different patients respond to pain differently, and this only compounds the problem of quantifying the pain and figuring out treatment for it. It was correct to assume that, since the patient was a junior football star who never had opioids or surgery before, his pain was going to be intense. To keep him calm and to prevent him from having stress reactions to pain in his post-op period, the decision was made to medicate with oral opioids. What started as a medical treatment post-surgery unfortunately turned into an addiction rather quickly for this patient. It was now four years removed from his surgery, and the patient was an emaciated, unkept, malodorous, homeless young man, who was concerned about finding another vein to get high.

The patient told David he had one vein on his lower leg, pointing to the large saphenous vein on his right leg, that he said he was saving for a special occasion. David inquired further, and the patient reported he was planning to use that vein over the holidays and New Year's and didn't want to blow it. He described all the places he tried to access veins after most of his peripheral veins were stripped and they no longer worked. Initially he tried on top of his foot and between his toes, then behind his knee, and ultimately (prior to injecting in his penis) between his lower eyeball and eyelid. David knew from school that heroin addicts try initially to hide their shooting up by injecting either right under their eye or between their toes in an effort to not get caught. The patient had four years of suffering and now had a penile infection.

David did the admission orders and called the on-call urologist. He made the patient NPO, meaning he could have nothing to eat or drink after midnight, and booked him for surgery the next day. The questions that loomed were these: Could they save the patient's penis? Would he need revisional surgeries and potentially implants? Would his penis be amputated the next day and a catheter placed?

David headed back to the resident lounge, shaking his head and wondering why we couldn't go back to opening psychiatric asylums and forced treatment facilities again. This patient had been arrested multiple times and lost his place to live and likely his family. During moments of insight, he was extremely depressed, and it was likely a psychiatric break or just the strong grip of his heroin addiction that lead to this masturbation with a cock ring (to engorge his veins) and then shooting up heroin.

David was in a daze, his mind running wild, when his beeper went off. He was almost to the resident lounge, so he took out his cell phone and returned the page. A nurse asked him to urgently come evaluate his patient Manuel. He went up to his room immediately and discovered the patient was having chest pains again, except this time the police were bedside, and the patient was handcuffed to his bed rails. Manuel denied taking any additional substances as he tried to grip his chest and breathe, but he appeared to be either intoxicated or having a panic attack. As the police read Manuel his Miranda rights, David noticed the scale was on his bedside table along with heroin in small bags—black tar—something David had never seen before. It dawned on David the patient was dealing drugs—in the hospital.

David walked out as the police went through the process of arresting Manuel, and he crouched down in the hallway, staring off in the distance. As he turned his head, he saw the young female heroin addict from downstairs in the emergency department. She went to turn into Manuel's room but saw the two police officers and immediately turned away and ran to the stairwell. David chased after her and caught up with her in the back stairway. He asked her if she knew the patient and what in the world was going on. Sobbing, the young lady admitted that Manuel was indeed a drug dealer in the hospital and that he also ran a prostitution ring in the hospital. This explained why he was a "frequent flyer" who was in and out of the hospital for chest pain and commonly known to visit the hospital.

He was collecting patients' welfare, retirement, and Social Security checks while feeding these sick (and often terminal), lonely patients both prostitutes and drugs. The young woman said she came to the hospital often to turn tricks set up by Manuel and was paid in heroin. However, she was recently getting less and less heroin and was concerned that one day it may be laced with a chemical to kill her when she injected. Her only payment was the prostitution drugs and rarely money, and there had been less business because the police presence had increased; she was convinced they were on to this game.

In addition, Manuel had developed a cocaine problem. She said that before meeting her boyfriend in the emergency department, she had brought crack cocaine to Manuel to free base in the room. Her boyfriend knew about and encouraged the prostitution so that they had money or heroin for both of them to get high. David asked the young woman if she would check into the emergency department as a patient and get clean. She refused and ran down the stairs crying.

David went to the nurses' station and put in new orders for Manuel, including a drug toxicology screen and chest pain work-up labs and imaging. Knowing it was only a cocaine reaction, he started to chart on the patient when his pager went off again.

This time it was security asking about another patient on his list, a post-operative patient from a foot amputation. He was known to have MRSA, C. diff, VRE (vancomycin resistant enterococcus)—a host of dangerous bacteria, or super bugs, particularly found in a hospital with immune-compromised patients. The security officer said the patient got heroin from a hospital dealer, and David knew exactly where he got it. The police came to question him, and he took off, hopping and running. David went to the elevators and down four floors to the patient's room. When he got off the elevator, numerous staff and police were looking at the floor. There was blood all over the floor from the patient's room to the stairwell.

The general surgeon had done a guillotine amputation and left the wound open to drain infection to get the site clean and free of bacteria before taking the patient back for a below-knee amputation closure. The patient could run, but not well.

The major issue was what to do when a patient with MRSA, C. diff, and VRE is bleeding and running around the hospital? Police caught the patient, and extra cleaning services staff were brought in with protective equipment to clean the entire floor.

David again shook his head. Having been an intern for six months, he was no longer surprised by occurrences like this. Prostitution and illicit drug sales and use, along with police intervention would continue long-term, and somewhere in that mix healthcare workers would be forced to be involved.

CHAPTER 12
It's a Pain

Robert enjoyed working with diabetic pain-medication seekers, essentially drugs addicts seeking opioids, particularly when it came to their feet. In this hospital almost 25 percent of emergency department visits involved the foot and ankle—likely the most injured body part in the United States. During this intern year, the hospital had patients with bullets in feet, dog bites to feet, cuts and scrapes on feet, and feet impaled with a car key, forks, nails from nail guns, pieces of wood, and the list goes on and on.

When the patients have uncontrolled or advanced diabetes and neuropathy has started, they no longer feel their feet. Of course, they can still have neuropathy pain—a strange occurrence of having no feeling in the skin or bones, but still having pain— which can be severe and debilitating, and which can lead to the mental expectation of pain.

Robert saw numerous patients admitted for either infections or traumas, such as those described above, who would ask for pain medicine. Every nurse and physician seem to record heart rate (pulse), respirations, temperature, blood pressure, oxygen level, height, weight, and, of course pain level. The hospital is for consumers now, not patients. The hospital systems want good reviews online, and many times they cater to patients instead of patient care. There is no objective way to measure pain. It's not uncommon to see open-heart surgery patients who require no post-operative pain medication, and then patients who have a surface laceration stitched in the emergency department who demand pain medication.

Consumer healthcare is mostly to blame for the opioid crisis. Physicians want to help patients, so when the patient says they're experiencing pain at a level of 10 out of 10, something must be done. Opioids can be used for this. Certainly, pharmaceutical companies and physicians have their share of blame in the current opioid crisis in America. However, consumer healthcare—or society at large—is just as much to blame. We've convinced people that they should have no pain, ever, which is not realistic. Pain is a mindset; if you come in prepared for it, you can handle it. If you come into pain not expecting any, then you can't handle that well. Every year we age we expect there to be more pain than the year prior, and if we have surgery or a trauma, we expect there to be some pain. There is no magical medication pill or intravenous fluid that will take away all the pain—mental or physical.

Robert had many patients who, when he woke them up from a sound sleep while making his hospital rounds, would tell him their pain was 10/10, even as they yawned and looked comfortable in bed. This would drive Robert to insanity as he expected 10/10 to be the worst thing imaginable—pain worse than death that shouldn't just be thrown around by patients. In a sick, twisted way, Robert enjoyed every minute of this in the diabetic foot population.

Pre-operative, the patient would have 10/10 pain and continue to take opioids. Sometimes pain management, which is the doctors and nurse practitioners dedicated to the pain medication specialty, both in hospital and outpatient, would have to be involved. Of course, the patient has neuropathy, and all the pain is simply in their head or nerve pain. Robert doesn't doubt that they feel it, but they're about to go to surgery and feel real pain, sometimes for the first time in their life. The patient goes from having a bone-exposed wound in their foot before surgery, saying how tough they are because they can handle this, to having surgery and curling up in the fetal position in pain.

Many times with foot procedures, the podiatrist and orthopedist who do these surgeries balance a tendon in the lower leg, such as the Achilles tendon, which is on the back of the heel and is commonly injured by athletes and weekend warriors alike. It's the biggest tendon in the body, and its power of pull can be decreased by lengthening. So, the diabetic with neuropathy doesn't feel the front of their foot being amputated, but they have complete feeling in their calf and have a ton of pain.

Robert couldn't keep his mouth shut with these patients. "How does it feel to really have pain?" he would ask with a sarcastic smirk at times.

Some patients would say that their pain was now a 20 out of 10 and get upset with the intern, cursing at him and asking for more pain medication. They built up a tolerance to opioids, so now they don't get any relief and have to have stronger doses, which leads down the rabbit hole to stronger drugs (even outside the hospital) and addiction. The body quickly becomes addicted, even if the patient doesn't enjoy the feeling of taking the medication. However, many patients tell Robert that they indeed didn't know real pain, and now their pain scale of 0 to 10 has shifted. They freely admit they were either pain-medication seekers before or confused by neuropathy or that they saw the condition of their foot as painful.

Although acting like a sadist, as if he were enjoying others in pain, Robert was actually educating many patients who turned around, adjusted their pain scale, and started to wean themselves from or get off opioids completely. Robert was responsible for countless patients realizing they were caught up in the opioid crisis with addiction and were able to turn their lives around.

For now, the physician continues to be tied to what the patient tells them, even if they know the patient is lying, and they have to treat them. As long as this physician-to-patient dynamic continues, there will be an opioid crisis, and doctors like Robert will continue to enjoy watching people in real pain and many times getting the satisfaction of helping them recover.

CHAPTER 13
Party Time

The nurse on the surgical floor frantically paged David regarding a patient who had barricaded her door. They needed a physician to talk to her. The patient was a disheveled, mid-30s female from the inner city who had come in for management of a pilon fracture (a fracture right above the ankle). She had a halo on that was set to be removed the next morning and then definitive hardware placed to fix the site. She was using crutches to ambulate and to keep the external fixator off the ground. The patient was rail thin, and David knew of her for two reasons: she had a boisterous, laughing personality, and she had a thing for one of the senior residents at the hospital.

Because this wasn't truly an emergency, David had taken his time getting to her floor. By the time he turned the corner, there were security, nursing staff, and administrators standing in the hallway and yelling through the door. The patient's door was shut, and she had indeed somehow barricaded the door. Since there was no lock on the door, the assumption was she used furniture to lock herself in. There was no other way into the room.

David noticed the stench of marijuana and smoke pouring out from under the door and realized she was hotboxing and laughing at them from inside the room. David had a good rapport with the patient from the orthopedic clinic, and since she had said it was nice to speak with him, he asked what it would take to get her to open the door.

"Get me that sugar doctor with the soul patch!" she replied.

While security was getting angrier and threatening to kick the door down, David started to laugh, knowing exactly which resident she wanted to see. By this time, more nurses had come around, and patients were starting to come out of their rooms. There was a strong odor of marijuana throughout the hallways.

Fortunately, the resident with the soul patch lived near the hospital. He was a senior resident who was the joke of the intern class because he acted cool but had a soul patch to cover up his insecurity and shyness. (You know the type: the guy at a party who talks to a girl and then just keeps talking and talking about how great he is until the girl loses interest—in other words, he was self-centered and not a closer.) As an intern class, they figured he had never kissed a real woman before.

So, the resident (later referred to as "Dr. Soul") showed up, walking down the hallway in jeans, a T-shirt, a leather jacket, and, of course, his soul patch on point. He said hello to the patient from outside the door. David could hear her hurrying on her crutches to the door and removing what turned out to be a small dresser. Then the door opened. The patient had been having a party of one, smoking marijuana and drinking a six-pack of beer, which she had finished. The patient said she was just trying to relax and live it up before undergoing anesthesia and surgery the next day.

Security and the police filled out a report but decided not to arrest the patient. The hospital didn't press charges for this reason: the patient claimed a different security guard sold her the marijuana and brought her the beer, which was never confirmed. However, a slim woman with a large external fixator in a hospital gown on crutches likely didn't leave the hospital and go get these items on her own. Perhaps there was a dealer who brought them to her, or perhaps she brought them from home initially; however, the beers had been cold, and there was no refrigerator in the room. She got them somehow, and the hospital wanted to avoid any of this getting out to the public.

The most amazing part of this encounter was how willing the resident was to come in to see the patient. He spent another 30 minutes with her, talking in her room. The interns thought if he was repulsive to all other women, perhaps having a woman who adored him was just what he needed.

At the end of the intern year, it came out that the resident was in a serious relationship with that patient. The resident no longer treated her and had informed the hospital's human resources department of this relationship. The resident is a lot calmer and nicer to everyone now, and it's assumed he's at least kissed a real woman.

CHAPTER 14
Heroines of Heroin

As you've already read during the intern year numerous teenagers and young adults came into the hospital with complications from heroin and other substance abuse. Certainly, the opioid epidemic has its grip on many parts of the country, but we forget this has been going on for decades in the inner city, though the media has now made it a priority since it has reached the suburbs.

Robert was on the house officer rotation, and the L&D (labor and delivery) unit was overcrowded and poorly staffed. The family practice residents were there to help cover deliveries when the OB/GYN residents weren't available, which was a great learning opportunity for those who wanted to be primary care physicians in a rural area.

Robert, however, was set on being a surgeon, so this was merely a nuisance for him unless he was able to see the C-sections. As the house officer, he was responding to postpartum problems and had to work with the addiction medicine physician who was a happy-go-lucky, self-described hippy. She was obviously brilliant, and she devoted her career to helping drug addicts. A woman in her early 50s, she had multiple colors in her hair and wore purple and blue, large-rim glasses. She was usually seen with coffee in hand and multiple papers and books/guides sticking out of her pockets. She was also very flirtatious, particularly with the male interns. Everyone knew she was more of hipster who thought she was 25 years old instead of a hippy.

Robert learned a lot about himself and about humility, grace, thankfulness, and tragedy during his time in the NICU (neonatal intensive care unit). At the hospital, the NICU was part of L&D, and once they were stable, the newborns (if they were able to live) would be transferred to a local children's hospital. Many of the babies in the NICU were born to heroin addicts, which meant they were born with an addiction and a need for opioids. These children had a small chance to survive and thrive in society; however, everyone deserves a chance, and many great people have been born to addicts and made a major impact in society.

The mothers and fathers of these children were restricted to minimal visits and were supervised by a team of staff and security because of a realistic fear they would leave with the children and harm them. Robert experienced addicts attempting to administer heroin to the newborns, thinking they were helping their children. Typically, there are arguments between families about custody of the newborn, or the parents are escorted by police because they're incarcerated. Animal studies have revealed horrible effects when infants are taken from their mother, so the hospital tries to expose the child to the mother when possible. However, heroin passes through the blood-brain barrier, meaning even breastfeeding can be dangerous if the mother is still using.

There were excellent volunteers and staff who spent time with these children. When the unit was overwhelmed, Robert had to watch the children himself. As any parent would understand, there's nothing worse than being unable to help your child when they're hurt. These small babies just born into this world were writhing in pain and crying for the opioids their body was used to. It's gut-wrenching to see someone you can't talk to and who doesn't understand go through withdrawal because of others' careless acts.

Many times, there were no mothers or fathers around. If the baby was lucky, perhaps there were grandparents who wanted to obtain custody. However, working with social services, Robert learned that, without the proper paperwork in place, which the heroin addict never had, it was tough to keep these children from their biological parents and the government system. Even if a grandparent was willing and ready to take custody, the child would have to become a ward of the state (put into the foster-child system) prior to the grandparents being granted custody. Although Robert had experienced academic challenges before with school, his previous experience did not prepare him for the stress and mental toll this rotation put on him.

Stress can come in many forms, and it amazed Robert how the staff handled this as it became normal to them. Robert was exhausted; he wasn't eating and felt nauseous most days. There were times when he would border on panic attacks going in to work on the children, as he wondered how bad the screaming and suffering would be or what type of argument he would get into with a mother that day. Given the walks down long hospital halls with minimal sleep and the stress of being an intern, plus a stressful daily experience in the NICU, at times the floor would shift/sway and he would feel off-balance. This was anxiety and borderline panic attacks. However, there was also great satisfaction with the daily work, and in the end, it made him a better physician.

CHAPTER 15
The Sugars

David was eager to start the morning rounds, and when a pleasant, moderately obese, African American, 72-year-old female came in with flu-like symptoms, he was assigned to this patient. Her blood work showed she was in DKA, which is diabetic ketoacidosis; her A1C was 12.3—much higher than normal. Knocking softly, David went into the patient's room. She had a large family, and there were times when over 30 people were there to visit. She was reported to make the best peach cobbler in the city.

"Good morning, Mrs. Barnett!" David said, walking to the patient's bedside. "How are you feeling?"

"Much better, honey," she replied.

David explained to the patient that her lab results came back, and now that they knew what was going on, they would get her feeling better soon. The patient was relieved.

David said, "Ma'am, you have diabetes." As an intern, David had never before told a patient they had diabetes, so he was very confused when the patient looked at him, smiled, and started crying tears of joy.

"Praise the good Lord," she said. "I thought you were going to tell me I had the sugars. The Lord done blessed me with this diabetes. The sugars will kill you!"

David's jaw dropped. He had been raised as an upper-middle working-class Caucasian from Florida and had spent his whole life around people with college or trade school educations. For the last 21 years, he had been in school—the last four around some of the brightest minds at a sought-after private medical school in the South. Nothing had prepared him for this conversation.

David stumbled to find the right words as tears welled up in his eyes and his thoughts flashed through what life must be like for this patient and how she saw the world differently than he did, with less formal education and different life experiences. How would he explain treating diabetes, a complex protocol, to this patient when she didn't even know the term? There was no preparation for the socioeconomic and educational challenges physicians faced when trying to have meaningful communication with patients in the hospital.

"Ma'am," David reported, "diabetes is 'the sugars.'" Not knowing how to explain anything else as he'd planned—he planned to explain the pathophysiology and treatment options—he was uncomfortable. So instead he just said, "We'll get you feeling better, and I'll see you later today."

David went straight to the bathroom and cried. He cared deeply about his patients and wasn't prepared for this encounter. After wiping away his tears, he left the bathroom, determined to start an outreach education program in the future on diabetes. This was a big jump for a surgical resident to do medicine rotations and plan for doing diabetes treatment in the future.

At table rounds that morning, David found his co-resident Robert. He told Robert the story, who shrugged off the comments, saying, "I just tell all my patients it's 'the sugars.' My family calls it 'the sugars,' so it's natural, I guess."

Robert had grown up poor, and the inner-city had hardened him in Section 8 housing with a single mother who was a nurse's aide, and his environment was a lot like the one in which Mrs. Barnett lived. Robert always said his mother wanted him to be a doctor more than anything else in the world, and that after retirement, he planned to start his real career. Robert explained that just because patients don't have the language doesn't mean they are not smart and savvy. Just as people can't talk to doctors, doctors have trouble talking to engineers and other professionals, as each profession has its own language.

David asked Robert, "How do you get through it mentally?"

Robert said, "Football, my man. That's the reason I'm here and that's how I continue to survive."

CHAPTER 16
Chasing the Blizzard

During our intern year we started covering an outlying community hospital (there was an agreement as they were in the same health system) because they needed help with coverage of on call shifts for surgery. In our facility there are surgical podiatrists who to our understanding do an additional three years of residency training to take hospital call and to do surgeries on feet and ankles. They also take infection cases, traumas, deformities, etc.

Robert was rotating through the orthopedic and podiatry service, and while he was sleeping at the Level 1 trauma center in the call room, his pager went off. He woke up like he had been shot out of a cannon and returned the call. It was the outlying small hospital requesting the foot service see a patient immediately. Robert said he would be there as soon as he was able, and he hung up and headed to his car.

On the 15-minute drive he called the day podiatry team who had handed him their list prior to the night call starting. The residents reported the patient he was going to see was post-op that day from having a transmetatarsal amputation (the front of his foot was cut off) due to a diabetic complication. The site was left open; no closure or partial closure was performed in surgery. Robert knew all too well this meant a bad infection had occurred; a bad infection can't be sewed up because any bacteria that remains will brew further. Leaving it open allows the site to drain; there would be plans to return later and perform the closure. This also meant there was a high bleeding risk.

While walking into the hospital, Robert got a call from the attending podiatrist who performed the patient's surgery only hours before. The attending, who was working his way up in administration at the main hospital and doing less clinical/surgical time, told Robert the entire story. The patient was in DKA, diabetic ketoacidosis, and he had known the patient for years as a noncompliant patient. Diabetic ketoacidosis, in short, is excess blood acids, or ketones, when there isn't enough insulin in the body and the blood sugar levels are severely elevated. The attending described this patient as having "cerebral neuropathy" (meaning he was numb between the ears and didn't do what he was supposed to do—he either had too low of an IQ or was too stubborn to listen to anyone). After surgery, the patient was told that he might need to go back into surgery the next day and was not allowed to eat.

Well, that didn't sit well with the patient, so he wheeled himself out of the hospital's front doors. When he was spotted on the security camera, they thought he was just going outside to smoke again. He wasn't. He called an Uber, and when the car pulled around, the patient positioned his IV pole and medications in the back seat, held his hospital gown around him, and got into the car. Security tried to track down the car, using the local police for assistance, but no one could find the patient.

Eventually, the police were called to the local Dairy Queen where the patient had passed out. The ice cream shop staff were frantic as he wouldn't wake up and was bleeding through his foot dressing, which was a no-brainer since the front of his foot bones, arteries, veins, nerves, ligaments, and tendons were exposed. The patient was in DKA and decided to eat ice cream. By all accounts his blood sugar was at least 600 or more and although barely functioning and near death he decide to raise his blood sugar more with ice-cream. The patient wasn't ignorant to DKA risk as he'd had this condition many times in the past. The police and EMS took him back to the hospital where the intake team were perplexed as no one knew the patient's name. He didn't have an ID on him; however, he was in a hospital gown and had an active IV pole with medications being administered.

Robert walked into the emergency department, and the doctor thanked him for getting there so quickly. He knew the backstory and could hear the patient yelling from the room, complaining about being held hostage and in jail. The emergency department physician had stabilized the patient and planned to readmit him to his room on the floor per the hospital medicine team.

The dressing was soaked with blood and clots. He had lost approximately 1,000 mL of blood. The patient was being transfused as his hemoglobin dropped while bleeding out at Dairy Queen. (Mind you, he was bacteremic—meaning bacteria in the bloodstream—with MRSA, methicillin resistant staphylococcus aureus, dangerous bacteria.) Robert first used a blood-pressure unit to make a tourniquet, then hemostats and sutures to tie off small arterial bleeders. He applied pressure with foam and thrombin to stop the oozing bleeding. Once the bleeding was controlled, a dressing was applied, and the tourniquet removed.

Robert told the patient how near death he was that night. The patient said he understood "he'd been to the mountaintop" and said he would try to be compliant but couldn't guarantee that.

He seemed to be oblivious about his condition. Because of his neuropathy, he felt no pain; he couldn't feel his foot being open or bleeding through his bones or other injuries. It was, for all intents and purposes, out of sight, out of mind.

Next, Robert documented the encounter, then called the attending back and told him the patient was stable at that time and was being transferred up to the floor for admission; he shouldn't hear from him again. Robert had removed the majority of the debris and dirt from the site and recommended a return to surgery the next day as initially planned. The patient was at a high risk of losing his leg and his life over the next couple days; however, the patient was still fired up and angry about his life-saving treatment being equal to jail. In the morning, the Behavioral Health team was set to evaluate the patient and deem whether or not he could make his own medical decisions.

Robert drove back to the Level 1 trauma center. He was looking forward to some sleep since his pager hadn't gone off again, which was rare for the Level 1 trauma call. He laughed to himself during the whole drive, thinking about the ice cream shop employees who didn't call 911 when a distraught, middle-aged, angry man walked into the restaurant before midnight wearing only a hospital gown, with his foot wrapped in bloodstained bandages and carrying an IV pole with an IV in his arm. They served him, and the man ate the ice cream, and no other customers or employees thought anything of this. When he lost consciousness, though, they finally called for help.

Robert continued to smile as he went back to sleep in the call room, thinking thankfully, *I won't have to see this patient again.* After sleeping for what felt like an eternity (in reality, only three hours), the pager went off again. It was the doctor in the emergency department of the Level 1 trauma center asking if he was covering the podiatry service. Robert said he was.

"You're not going to believe this patient," the emergency doctor told him. "It's got to be the most noncompliant patient I've seen." Then the doctor proceeded to tell him the patient was found walking on the side of the highway, wearing a hospital gown and with an IV pole. From all accounts he'd walked a few miles and was bleeding through a foot dressing.

"Let me guess," Robert said, "he had a transmetatarsal amputation yesterday, and the attending emergency department physician sounded like he was surprised."

"Yes! That's the patient!"

"I saw him a few hours ago," Robert said. "I'll be right down."

Robert was less urgent this time. He was more annoyed that an on-call night in which he could have had some sleep had turned into chasing this noncompliant, uneducated, mad-at-the-world diabetic neuropathic for his foot wound. As he pulled back the curtain in the emergency department room, he saw the same patient—who was now dirty and sweating—with a saturated dressing he had put on only a few hours earlier. Robert asked what happened.

"I just couldn't stay there, man," the patient replied. "I asked the cops and ambulance that picked me up to take me to this hospital." The police were outside his door.

The plan was to admit him to the floor and ask behavioral health to see him in the morning with plans to "pink slip" the patient, a term that means take their shoes, belt, and anything else they could use to hurt themselves, give them a special gown that will enable all hospital employees to see them as a psychiatric patient, and put them on a psychiatric hold.

Fortunately, there was less blood this time since the sutures had held the arterial bleeders. Arterial bleeding will cause pulsatile bleeding; in other words, every time the heart beats, the blood squirts with enough force (based on blood pressure) to fly across the room. This was all vein blood now, which was just oozing.

Robert opened the site and used a cautery tool to burn the veins. He soaked gauze in thrombin and applied a bulky pressure dressing to the wound so that it wouldn't bleed. Of course, it was 3:00 a.m., and he had to wake up the attending physician again to tell him what happened. The doctor couldn't wrap his head around the patient's behavior. They talked about using the same IV line as again he still had his pole with him and was medications. They changed the plans and decided to take the patient to surgery at the current hospital in a few hours for washout and debridement. Again, the patient didn't seem to notice his foot was wide open and bleeding.

Heading back to the on-call room, Robert got into the elevator and ran into another resident on call for the medicine team. He told him the story, and they shook their heads. Only in residency will you see this; they couldn't believe how much their world had changed since they began working with "the public" now that they were out of school. Their sleepless nights wouldn't last, but the stories sure would.

"At least that's the last time I have to see this patient," Robert told the other resident. After documentation, he went upstairs to sleep for a couple hours before turning over the list of patients to the day team and heading on to his rotation for the day. He was currently on vascular surgery, so he prepared to remain (tired) at work until he got to go home around 5:00 p.m.

He woke up at 6:00 a.m., changed his scrubs, reviewed the list, and updated everything on the computer with plans to hand off the list. While walking to the morning conference room to give his report, thinking about how to present the case, his pager went off again. Robert was upset; he was supposed to be off call and not receiving calls from the operator after 6:00 a.m. It was 6:02 a.m. He thought about ignoring the call and having them call the other intern on call for the day; instead, he returned the call.

The operator said an emergency department attending from another hospital (and actually another health system) in the city wanted to speak with him.

"I have a patient who says you treated him at two hospitals overnight," said the ED attending.

"What?!" yelled Robert.

"Yeah," said the attending, "the patient left the Level 1 trauma center out a back stairwell. Apparently, this time he removed his IV line himself. He held pressure on his arm and went outside to the busy city street and hailed a cab. The cab driver thought it was strange that he was in an odd-colored hospital gown. The patient apparently asked to be taken home, but five minutes into the ride he passed out—of course, still bleeding from the foot and with uncontrolled blood glucose. The taxi driver called the police and drove him here."

"I'm sorry," Robert said. "We don't cover call at your hospital. Someone else will need to take over the patient care."

And that was the end of the night Robert chased a patient around town. He did have some friends that worked as residents at the other hospital, so later that night he called one of them, Ethan, who was on the surgery service. They had been in medical school together, and Ethan thanked Robert sarcastically for sending over his patient. The patient went right to the operating room, received a below-knee amputation, and was in restraints in the psychiatric ward. The patient would have kept all his foot except for the front of it if he had just stayed put and been compliant.

The patient had escaped the psychiatric hold and the police at the Level 1 trauma center where Robert worked, which bought him restraints and a full lockdown in a psychiatric ward at the new hospital.

Shaking his head, Robert told Ethan, "Well, at least I know I won't see him anymore because he can't get up and walk out without a leg!"

In a stressful, sleep-deprived night, only laughter can get you through, and Robert thought, *One day, I'll be telling my kids and grandkids about this night.*

After being on for a 36-hour shift, it was time for Robert to sleep … and to wonder if it was just a dream.

CHAPTER 17
Accountability

David looked over his list in the morning. There was an uninsured patient with a leg abscess who was also in diabetic ketoacidosis, which is a dangerous condition in uncontrolled or ill diabetics. In the community, this is commonly referred to as a diabetic coma.

David reviewed the labs and was scanning through them quickly when he suddenly stopped and said, "Damn! Is this a mistake?" he asked the resident on the service. The resident explained it wasn't a mistake; it was simply a high value. The patient's HgbA1c was over 21. The HgbA1c is a measurement of glucose on hemoglobin in diabetics and gives roughly a three-month measurement of diabetic control—or, in this case, lack of control.

To put this in perspective, an A1c of 21 is equivalent to an average glucose measured at any time of day of 556. Most people at this level can't function physically or metabolically; however, this patient had been living for the past three months at this level.

The patient was 71-year-old gentlemen with a long white beard. He was bald on top but had a ponytail. He had poor dentition and was wide awake (not comatose) when David saw him. David prepared him for the leg-abscess incision and drainage for surgery, explaining to the patient that the surgery site would likely not heal and would have continued infection. He said the patient may even need an amputation; however, at the patient's glucose level, even an amputation was likely not to heal.

The patient was not fazed by this conversation. He reported knowing he was diabetic and that he had ignored it—quite the rationalization with that A1c level. He was at risk of dying with surgery as well.

The surgery was successful, and post-operative his glucose was starting to improve into the 400s and occasional 300s. The plans were for David to see the patient in the resident teaching clinic for post-op follow-up, given that he had no insurance. David worked hard with the social workers to get the patient medications for free, including the insulin he would need.

The patient refused the help. "I know what caused this, and I'll take care of it!" he told David. The third day post-op, the patient left AMA—against medical advice—which is when the patient signs out, saying they know the risks, and leaves. This is not just walking out.

Patients often feel powerless and will try to take control of the situation, which is both unfortunate and costly. An example of this is when a patient has a surgery scheduled for 2:00 p.m. that they desperately need, and they have not been able to eat or drink since midnight. The patient will say, "The doctor needs to do this surgery sooner, or I'm going to start eating and drinking."

The overworked surgeon typically responds, "Great, let the patient eat and drink so I can cancel and do the case later."

David once had a patient threaten to and then eat on a Thursday because the patient didn't want to wait. They were sure the attending surgeon would care enough and would do the surgery at 7:00 a.m. the next day—the first surgery of the day. The busy surgeon, who was operating at many hospitals in the system, said it was okay and did indeed take him back to surgery at 7:00 a.m.—the following Thursday. The patient created a costly mistake for the hospital, insurance, and mostly to the patient by delaying care. (This was an urgent but not emergent surgery and so was able to wait a week.)

About four months after David's 21 HgbA1c patient left AMA, David was working the busy inner-city surgery resident training clinic. He saw the name of the patient with the super-high A1c pop up on the computer. To David's shock, he walked into the room and saw a perfectly healed incision and drainage site with minimal scarring. (Remember, the last time he saw the leg, it was still open and being packed.) The patient was in no pain, but David thought that was related to neuropathy.

He ordered a new A1c and asked the patient to stay longer in the clinic and wait for the lab result to finalize, and the patient agreed. David saw the remainder of the clinic patients, and then went back into the patient's room. The patient had told David he came in thinking he should finally follow up (months later). He also told David he didn't take the insulin or other medication prescribed.

David looked at the lab results in the patient's chart, and there it was: HgbA1c of 5.8.

David went into the room and said, "Sir, you said you knew what was causing the diabetes and would take care of it, but how did you do it?"

The patient said, "That's easy. All my diet consisted of were Little Debbie cakes and sweet wine!"

Just like that, the patient was four months sober, and he hadn't had to go to the hospital for withdrawal from alcohol, which was amazing in itself. He seemed upbeat and happy. He told David that the surgery cured his taste for alcohol and he was thankful. His life was turned around.

Everything David knew of alcoholics and being a physician was turned upside down.

CHAPTER 18
Call the Toe Truck

During the intern year there was a wave of lawn mower versus foot and leg injuries as the winter weather melted away to a beautiful spring. Apparently, this was a common occurrence, but one we weren't exposed to in medical school in trauma classes or on rotations in suburban hospitals. These high-energy, complex traumas are typically brought to the Level 1 trauma center.

The scenario usually plays out such that a patient gets intoxicated or distracted and they run themselves over with the auto-propelled lawn mower, push mower, weed trimmer, or— worse yet—the riding mower. We all learned that a large majority of patients like to mow their yard with a beer in hand and flip-flops on. It's hot and sunny and they're not used to it, and injuries occur.

It was common for family and friends in the trauma bay to tell us that, right before the injury occurred, the patient said, "Hold my beer, watch this!" (This applies to yard injuries, falls from heights, high-energy crashes, and so on.)

Robert was covering the Saturday shift over Memorial Day weekend at the hospital as the house officer. (Many interns had requested and actually been granted a vacation weekend.) Robert had numerous pagers on his waist as he had the on-call pager as well as all the vacationing interns' pagers, in case there were any calls for them. Pagers, although antiquated, work better than cell phones from a coverage standpoint because you're not going to miss a page. However, pagers have a short range, and if you travel out of the region, they typically don't work.

It had been a quiet holiday so far, which put a pit in Robert's stomach because he knew it was only a matter of time before traumas started coming in. It was one of the first warm, sunny days of the year, and a holiday weekend on top of it. He was prepared for motorcycle crashes, injuries such as burns from grilling food, street fights, alcohol-related injuries, etc. Little did he know this was going to be lawn-mower day.

The first patient came by EMS from an hour away. He was a non-intoxicated, middle-aged truck driver who had been mowing his 10-acre property. He was found by his father in the field when he didn't answer a phone call (fortunately his father lived next door). The father—a 70-year-old mountain of a man with hands like sandpaper and darkened, sunken eyes—was in the emergency department bay with his son. The father had a weathered look likely gained from a life of manual labor and farming. He had the look of a former body builder, and thankfully for the patient, he was strong as an ox.

The patient had been mowing along a hillside when the riding mower tipped over. The mower was equipped with a switch meant to turn off the mower deck once you rise from the seat, but this was truly a freak accident as he didn't come off the seat because it happened so quickly. There he lay in the field with the lawnmower on its side and him pinned under the mower. The blades only stopped because the strong tibia (the lower leg bone) kept them from moving, causing the mower engine to fail.

Significant blood loss had occurred because of an arterial injury, and although farm soil and lakes are about as dirty as you can get from an infection standpoint, at that time, infection wasn't the concern. The priority was to stop the bleeding. With heaven-sent strength, his father lifted the riding mower off his son, and then he pulled off his belt and made a tourniquet below the knee. Next, the 70-year-old man threw his 245-pound son over his shoulder in a fireman's carry and headed to the house. Once there, he called 911. There was additional bleeding, and he applied pressure and put ice around the leg using a makeshift splint with reduction he built using two pieces of wood and some ties.

When he arrived to the trauma bay, Robert saw a man whose lower leg was full of debris, grass, and dirt. He irrigated the site, and the patient didn't seem to be in pain, probably due to both shock and nerve injury—he couldn't feel what was happening. Wet dressing was applied, and the trauma attending was already in the room. They headed for the operating room where the patient was to undergo the first of many surgeries to attempt to salvage his limb.

In the operating room, the leg was washed out and debrided. An external fixator (a mechanism where pins are placed in the bone and attached to rings or rods like an erector set) was placed. Healing from this injury would involve multiple specialties and numerous procedures with an extensive stay in a nursing home—essentially a heroic effort.

The patient lived, and by the end of the intern year, he still had his leg. Of course, this was going to be a chronic-pain situation, and it would never be a fully functional limb again. It would require bracing; however, for an over-the-road truck driver, he needed the limb—brace or not—to continue working.

Studies have been performed looking at the costs involved in the trauma or diabetic-infection setting when it comes to salvaging a lower extremity versus amputating it. From a financial standpoint, it's more affordable to primarily amputate; it's only one surgery and there are fewer risks of infection, chronic pain, and other complications. However, explaining that to a middle-aged father of two girls who drives a truck for a living is a different story. In addition, there are other studies that show an increase in mortality with lower-limb amputation, so it's still debated medically.

After the case, Robert was walking to the cafeteria when another page came through from the emergency department. He hadn't eaten or had a drink of water in about 20 hours, so he debated not returning the page. *They're going to keep calling*, he thought, so he called from the cafeteria phone.

"We have a lawnmower versus foot this time," said the emergency department attending, "and the patient's en route from three hours away via helicopter. Anticipate landing in five minutes."

Robert scarfed a piece of cold pepperoni pizza, then downed a bottle water while walking to the emergency department.

When he entered the trauma bay, Robert heard a lot of commotion surrounding a screaming, angry patient. The helicopter pilot and flight nurses were trying to calm the patient as they gave their report to the trauma-bay team. He was 25 years old with three young children and a wife back home. He lived on a farm, approximately 100 miles away from our Level 1 trauma center.

"If you all can just reattach my toe, I'd like to head back home!" the patient was screaming.

The patient had been mowing with an automatic push mower while wearing flip-flops and was backing up, forgetting the pile of bricks he had left in the yard that the grass had overgrown. As he backed up, with the mower in one hand and a Natural Light in the other, he tripped, and the mower went over the top of his right foot—a clean cut at the base where the big toe meets the foot. Initially he grabbed the toe and tried to keep mowing, but there was too much blood loss. His wife saw him sitting on the ground, holding his bleeding foot, and called 911 before running out to help.

The patient was young, and because of that and the fact that he had a good cardiac reserve, he could handle the significant blood loss better than an older patient. The patient's wife had the toe, which she had thrown on ice in a Ziplock bag, and the patient requested immediate surgery for his toe to be put back on. He did need emergency surgery—to decrease the risk of infection and to clean out the debris and grass from inside his foot. There was the potential for multiple future surgeries to prevent below-knee amputation. However, there was no surgery to save his toe.

As Robert explained this to the patient, he asked if his thumb could be used in place of his toe or—better yet—he wondered if he could get a cadaver toe. The patient said he had seen a story from Asia where they had used a patient's big toe in place of his thumb when a laborer had a similar accident on their hand. Robert explained to the patient that due to the risk of the surgery and repairing blood vessels and nerves that size, it was not a good idea. It would likely lead to rejection, further infection, and more pain and complications.

The patient was given intravenous pain medication as his adrenaline slowed and the pain set in. Robert explained to the calming patient that the toe was gone and that certainly no one would be willing to take this young father's thumb to recreate a toe. The patient was concerned about how his foot would look in the summer at the pool and while wearing sandals. Robert reassured him that silicon toes and foot prosthetics exist, and no one would know the difference. He would still be able to chase his kids. Plus, no surgeon in their right mind would remove a thumb, which by all accounts is more important than a big toe.

Prior to his arrival at the hospital, the flight team and paramedics had used silver nitrate sticks, pressure, and hemostat clamps to get the base of the big toe to stop bleeding. Then the patient received tetanus updates, IV antibiotics, and surgery for amputation with revision of the base of the toe. He was transfused blood and survived.

Of course, he wanted to keep his toe when he left the hospital, so he took it home. He told the trauma team he wanted to see if the toe could be gold plated for a necklace or if it could be embalmed to keep on his mantle. This is common to hear from amputees, and Robert often wondered how many people out there still had their amputated toe or body part. We always suggested that patients have a burial for the lost limb—but not a lost life. A few patients, likely based on cultural or religious reasons, have kept the limb to be buried with them whenever they die.

CHAPTER 19
Don't Let Sleeping Drunks Lie

A 50-year-old alcoholic patient was brought into the emergency department by his angry wife at about 7:30 in the morning, a couple days before Christmas, and Robert was on house officer. The patient was in severe pain, and his legs were dusky, gray, and darkening by the minute. The wife was arguing with the husband, so it was hard for Robert to focus the patient so that they could discuss what happened.

The patient didn't want to give his history; he just said he used to drink alcohol. Robert asked what he meant, and the patient said, laughing, "I used to drink alcohol. I still do, but I used to too!" The wife got upset when she heard this and ran out of the room.

Although the patient didn't realize it yet, he had gangrene of his legs from frostbite. Many times, frostbite (and what we call chilblains) can be healed with rewarming, antibiotics, tetanus, and sometimes vascular intervention. However, this patient was too far gone. Each year around the wintertime, the hospital sees an increase in the number of patients, who are usually homeless, admitted with frostbite. However, this patient was affluent and lived in the suburbs. He didn't fit the picture. He had sensation to his feet and no neuropathy or other medical issues.

The patient finally broke down and told Robert he had a sports gambling problem and a drinking problem. The night before, he was betting and losing, and at about 10:00 p.m. he stepped outside on the front porch to call his bookie. Of course, it was snowing and 15 degrees, and he was in flip-flops, shorts, and a T-shirt. He walked over to his car; he was worked up and expecting a quick phone call to get more money fronted.

That was the last thing he remembered. Apparently, on his way to the stairs of the front porch, he lost consciousness from intoxication. There he lay in the cold (it did get down to single digits Fahrenheit last night) for approximately eight hours. His wife and children had gone to bed, and because he usually stayed up in the basement "man cave" to watch sports until well after midnight, they didn't think anything of it when he didn't come to bed. (Many times, he would pass out drunk in his recliner in the basement.) However, the next morning, the wife couldn't find the patient in the basement, so the kids looked outside; there he was, facedown in the snow, still in a T-shirt, shorts, and sandals.

The family feared he was dead; however, he was awake and starting to sober up. The wife put him and the kids in the minivan and headed to urgent care where he was seen by a triage nurse and immediately sent to the hospital. The patient's pain started to increase as he was not getting blood flow to his feet. Gangrene had set in with the frostbite injury, and there was no turning back.

Talking to Robert, the patient went on and on about his high school football glory days, his career, sports, and drinking. Robert couldn't get a word in, so he just let the patient do his nervous talking while Robert thought that last night, this patient's greatest stress was losing on a sports bet; he must be overwhelmed now.

After about 20 minutes of the patient rambling on and telling Robert how great he was, Robert said, "You don't want to hear this, and neither do I want to tell you this, but I'm consenting you for surgery to have both your legs amputated below the knee." Robert told him he was beyond vascular repair and hyperbarics (an oxygen-chamber treatment used for patients with vascular compromise, wounds, bone infection, and the bends from diving).

The patient broke into tears, but he consented. Taking the legs saved his life. He stayed in the hospital and underwent withdrawal from alcohol and survived. He went on to a rehab center and apparently is doing well now. Amazingly, he stopped by at the end of the year; he was working to get out of a wheelchair and walk with a brace and wheeled walker. His wife and children were by his side.

His wife made a comment that has stuck with Robert to this day: "He lost his legs, and we found our husband and our father. The frostbite gangrene was the best thing that ever happened to this family."

Perhaps we all just need a perspective reset.

CHAPTER 20
Life Happens Fast

Robert was covering orthopedic trauma call on Sunday night, typically the slowest night for trauma call at this Level 1 hospital. Although any night can be unpredictable, traumas seem to occur most frequently Thursday through Saturday nights when people are out and about and intoxicated. Regardless, the summer was coming to a close, and fewer traumas had been seen in the emergency department.

It's not uncommon for the intern to be in charge of the service on a Sunday night. However, this was a rare Sunday night in which a locum (a locum is a temporarily employed doctor) from another hospital in town was on call for orthopedic trauma, though he was not expecting to have to come in. He was a young, total joint surgeon looking for extra cash from the hospital system, and he agreed to take the orthopedic trauma call shift; after all, he had been well trained in trauma during residency. (Most specialists in orthopedics, although trained on the entire body, only want to deal with their area of specialization and not take a general orthopedic trauma call.)

This locum attending was on call because the hospital orthopedic trauma surgeons, who were typically on call, were at a national conference where many of them were speaking. The issue with this was the fellows (the physicians who are done with residency and who are getting extra training in orthopedic trauma) were attending the conference too. So, there was Robert, nervous about being the only one to run the service for the hospital and afraid to call the total joint surgeon who he thought didn't really want to be bothered.

All was quiet, and Robert was sitting in the residency lounge checking charts and watching baseball on television. He was joking around with some of the other interns and residents and had just lost a game of billiards (there was an old pool table in their lounge near the on-call rooms) when he heard the announcement through the speakers that two Level 1 traumas would be arriving by helicopter in the trauma bays in 10 minutes. Robert scrambled for his pager and ID badge and headed out the door. Taking deep breaths, he thought about the fact that Level 1 is the highest, most at-risk level, and they may already be dead.

Perhaps there are no orthopedic injuries, he thought.

When Robert pulled the curtain back and walked into the trauma bay, he wasn't ready for what he saw: an 18-year-old man and a 17-year-old girl with severe trauma mostly to their extremities as well as internal injuries being managed by the general surgery trauma team. Robert was in shock himself as he slowly drifted toward the wall and grabbed the phone. He called the orthopedist on call, the total joint surgeon, and though he was willing to come in and help, he was about 30 minutes out. Robert's heart was in his throat.

First, he walked over to the young man whose right arm was severed below the elbow and hanging loosely by a couple tendons and some nerves and vessels. It looked like a ham you'd find at the butcher shop. His face was swollen, his eyes sunken, and there was bruising and obvious head injury. The neurosurgeon was evaluating him. Both his ankles were broken, and the right one was an open fracture. His pelvis appeared appropriate, and the emergency department attending and general surgery trauma attending were checking other sites for trauma.

The patient was coherent enough to be yelling in pain, but he was obviously in shock. Robert felt comfortable reducing and splinting the ankles and stabilizing the patient for the CT scanner. The right arm was placed in a splint and reduced as best as possible with saline-soaked gauze and fiberglass splinting with padding. The vessels in the fingers were somehow intact, and the fingers were warm; however, there was no function with likely nerve damage. This was why the patient wasn't guarding when moving the arm; he couldn't feel and likely would never regain function of his arm and hand.

As the young man was wheeled emergently to the CT scanner, Robert turned to look at the 17-year-old girl. The other emergency department physician and general surgery trauma surgeon were looking at her, examining the extent of her injuries. Portable X-rays were being taken. She was badly injured and came in and out of consciousness. She was also perfect. It turns out she was the beauty queen of a small town outside the city and a bright, adored young woman.

Robert started his survey as they cut off the remainder of her clothes, including matching bra and panties. The young girl's body was perfect, her skin supple and flawless. Her hair and makeup were done for a night out with her date. Robert looked past her natural C-cup breast and runway strip of pubic hair like a well-trained robot looking for injuries and caring for her. It wasn't until afterwards that he started to immerse himself into what the patient's life used to be.

Only thirty minutes ago this was a seemingly flawless 17-year-old girl, beauty queen, the pride of her family and parents as it turns out she was ranked #1 in her class academically, and she was lusted after by many teenage boys and young men. However, that was 30 minutes ago. Now her body wasn't perfect, and if she lived, she would spend the next 60 or more years in chronic pain—in hell—and deal with depths of depression and anxiety that most people will never face. She was a train wreck of orthopedic injuries, but fortunately, she did not have any head trauma on evaluation. She just had trauma everywhere else.

This hospital typically diverted traumas under 18 years old to the nationally acclaimed children's hospital in the same city. However, because they were both in the accident, both were brought there. Robert's jaw dropped when the portable films started to come in. The following is a breakdown of the injuries sustained by the teenage girl. Remember at that time Robert was the only person on the orthopedic trauma service, and the attending was driving in. He was in over his head; less than 6 months ago, he was still a medical student.

Her fractures included: talus (bottom bone of the ankle) on the right side; ankle fractures on both sides with the left higher at tibia-fibula than the right at the ankle joint; both femurs; pelvis; multiple ribs; left humerus, which was shattered; left wrist fracture; right collar bone; and a couple lumbar-level spine fractures. There were also multiple contusions and abrasions. The only thing spared was the right-upper extremity, except that her right hand was fractured throughout with open metacarpals. There she lay—a beautiful young torso with mangled extremities.

Robert knew the pelvis needed to be decompressed with the fracture, so he stabilized all the affected extremities as best he could with splints and then flew down the stairs to the basement of the hospital. The basement contains, as many hospitals do, a fenced-in, locked room holding what looks like torture equipment hanging everywhere. This is where all the equipment for traction is held: weights, pulley systems, chains, wires, counterweights, boards, etc. Picture a rusted hardware shop covered by a fence and secured with a door and a lock. Robert fumbled through the lock's combination and grabbed essentials. Although he struggled to carry everything by himself, including the offsetting weights and frames to add to the bed, he made it back to the trauma bay.

When he arrived, Robert saw the orthopedic attending on call was there with the young female patient, who was about to undergo at least 12 hours or more of surgery and needed to have stable fixation. Robert breathed a sigh of relief and expected gratitude from the surgeon, who should have been in the attending call room and not at home 30 minutes away. Robert was inexperienced, but he wanted to go into orthopedic trauma and prided himself on his knowledge base in this subject. Unfortunately, the orthopedic attending belittled him about the work he had done.

Robert told the attending to pin the patient and told him how to hang the pulley system. The attending scoffed, and Robert realized the unfortunate truth for the patient and himself: The attending had come from a slow-paced residency program, spending time at only a Level 2 trauma center; he had never had to deal with Level 1 trauma. Then his fellowship was all outpatient elective surgeries, not emergencies. Robert pushed past the attending and went to work, shaking his head as he realized the tongue-lashing he'd just received was the attending's defense mechanism.

So Robert, the intern, used a cordless driver that grasps a large, threaded, self-cutting pin and drives it through the young woman's legs and feet. Mind you, she was awake—or at least conscious—and in significant pain. The conscious sedation was given to her after her family arrived to sign consents. (Of course, there is implied consent in a trauma situation until proven otherwise.) Robert drove the pins, hooked up the rope and wire systems, added the frame to the bed and then the pulleys, and started adding weights. The patient groaned and tensed, even with sedation. Weights were added one at a time from the foot of the bed until the legs were pulled so hard the pelvis fracture gave and started to reduce and decrease pressure on the site. Although this may seem barbaric, it's the only way to hold reduction until surgery.

Towards the end, the patient's parents came into the trauma bay and started crying and hugging their daughter. She was braced, including her head and neck, and could only speak with them briefly. She was stabilized overnight, and one of the head orthopedic trauma surgeons at a competing hospital willingly accepted the patient as a transfer. Of course, the head of orthopedic trauma at Robert's hospital had to call from the conference and explain to the physician at the other hospital that no one equipped to handle the case was readily available. Robert knew residents at the other hospital and followed up with them regarding the patient's outcome.

It turned out the 18-year-old man was a professional motocross driver, a local legend in his town; he even competed on ESPN events. He also worked as a mechanic, meaning he had spent thousands of hours on a motorcycle in addition to driving other vehicles on and off-road. In other words, even though he was young, he was an experienced driver and in great shape. He was a proclaimed Christian and didn't use alcohol or drugs.

After meeting in a youth group at their church, this was the young couple's third date. Although she was picked up on a motorcycle, her parents weren't concerned because he was such a good driver and really cared about their daughter.

Come to find out, the couple had been stopped on the motorcycle at a stop sign on a country road. The young man was not wearing a helmet because he had given it to her. An old Cutlass sedan came flying around the corner, out of its right lane, and hit the stopped motorcycle at more than 65 mph. Authorities estimated the couple were thrown somewhere between 40 and 50 feet in the air before landing on the concrete on the opposite side of the road.

Fortunately, there was someone in an SUV opposite the motorcycle at the stop sign, facing them, who witnessed this. The sedan driver was stumbling drunk and thought he hit a deer until he had sobered up in jail and was told what he'd done. He obviously should not have been driving that night; he had been drinking all day and chose to drive to a friend's house to get more alcohol on a Sunday night.

The drunk driver had five previous DUIs—yes, five—in the past 20 years. He did not have a license or insurance. He was uninjured, though hopefully he will spend the majority of the remainder of his life in jail or on house arrest so that he can't hurt anyone else.

The young man survived; however, he had severe brain damage. He will spend the rest of his life in an extended-care facility unable to care for himself, the expenses for which will be covered by government-payer insurance given the drunk driver had no insurance. Remarkably the young girl lived and had multiple surgeries over the year to save her extremities. She is in chronic pain, which keeps her from holding down a job or maintaining relationships. She relies on oral opioids when awake due to the pain and likely will endure numerous additional surgeries in her lifetime to maintain this independence. However, she has made the most of this and has become a well-known speaker, discussing that night at high schools, colleges, and other places young people attend, telling them the real-life horror stories of drinking and driving.

Robert knows that the only reason she lived was because of his efforts that night. He's proud of her functional level but saddened by a perfect life turned to daily hell. It's said that things happen for a reason, but if you spend too much time in the trauma bay at the hospital, you start to question your understanding of this and of faith. Certainly, the trauma bay lights shined brighter that night, and a higher power guided an inexperienced Robert to help this patient.

CHAPTER 21
Cost Saving

On the top floor of the hospital, Samantha was in the gym, shooting basketball after doing a cardio workout on the rowing machine, when she was paged to the emergency department. She returned the call, panting and trying to catch her breath. The emergency department attending told her they had a Level 1 trauma—two teenage girls with multiple blunt-force injuries. It was a hot summer night, and Samantha could only imagine what she was walking into. Were these girls injured at a backyard BBQ, a concert, a festival …?

Samantha wiped herself down, threw on some scrubs, and headed to the elevators. In the emergency department, she went to the trauma bay and found the two badly bruised, beaten-up, 17-year-old girls. Based on the severity of the injuries, she initially thought it was gang violence, then she noticed they were well dressed and thought they might be from the affluent suburbs. Indeed, they had been best friends since beginning kindergarten in a Catholic school, and now attended a nationally ranked Catholic high school in the city.

As the staff cut their clothes off and started imaging with portable X-rays, Samantha began her full-body survey. Except for some forefoot lacerations, all the injuries appeared to be from blunt force. There were extremity fractures, but most concerning was the potential for internal bleeding. The young females were deteriorating, so the closed fractures were reduced and splinted.

The best friends each headed to the CT scanner and then to surgery at the same time, with a second trauma attending surgeon (in addition to the one on call), plus the team of staff for another operating room. The girls had been together since kindergarten and were now heading to adjacent operating rooms. At this point both were intubated and unconscious.

Samantha went to meet the parents with the trauma fellows in the lobby and brought them into a room. The good news, Samantha told the parents, was that the girls were alive. The bad news was that they had to have exploratory, open-abdominal surgery to stop the source of the bleeding and likely remove each patient's spleen. The families agreed with the plan; however, the mothers were focused and crying. The fathers of the patients seemed distracted and were steaming mad having their own conversation.

Patients often try to lie about their injuries—even in the trauma bay as their life hangs in the balance. Human beings don't like to admit to embarrassing stories. For instance, only a week prior, Samantha had seen patients who were victims of a collision between an 18-wheeler semitruck and other cars, which caused multiple traumas, although all the patients were alive when they arrived at the hospital.

The truck driver (or logistics professional, as he called himself) had lost focus on the road and ended up jack-knifing (when the trailer swings to the level of the front of the truck—imagine swinging a large baseball bat and the other cars and people are the baseball). As the patient was lying on the trauma bay table and his clothes were being cut off, he was fighting Samantha and the staff. Although his strength was limited due to blood loss and shock, he was fighting to remove a shoelace he had fashioned around his erect penis and testicles before the staff could see. It was obvious to the staff what was going on, and he was making excuses for this. It was no wonder he lost focus. Unfortunately, he didn't go down without swinging. The staff couldn't calm him down, and he expired shortly after in the operating room—a celestial discharge while holding his package.

For the current trauma, the fathers of the teenage girls told Samantha how the girls' injuries occurred. It was the most innocent teenage story, and yet one that made Samantha scratch her head and wonder if youth really is wasted on the young. The girls went to a bonfire party at the lake with friends, including their two boyfriends. (The fathers were not pleased that the girls were dating inner-city boys; they were public-school kids and not from an affluent family.)

A festival was being held near the lake that sounded like a lot of fun; it offered carnival-type games, livestock shows, live music and entertainment, and a demolition derby. The double-dating teenagers decided to head for the derby and found out from friends that the fee to get into the derby was two dollars for each person in the car. (Mind you, the teenagers—both boys and girls—were intoxicated and not used to drinking and driving. And no, there wasn't a car wreck.) About a half mile outside the entrance to the demolition derby, they pulled the car over, and the girls got into the trunk. (This was an old sedan that lacked any handle to open the trunk from the inside.)

The two teenage boys shut the trunk, got into the car, and drove slowly for the next half mile into the festival entrance, saving four dollars by having the girls in the trunk. As they pulled up to the derby, they saw some high school friends on the way and were talking through the windows. Meanwhile, the demolition derby started, which was incredibly noisy. The teenagers had never been to a demolition derby and were in awe at the power, the smell of exhaust, and the yelling crowd, not to mention the loud grinding sounds of steel on steel.

In their distraction, the boys forgot about the girls in the trunk and ran over to watch the action. They didn't think anything about the girls; they were just intoxicated teenage boys staring at cars deliberately wrecking into each other. After about an hour (and, of course, drinking some additional alcohol with their friends) they decided to head back to the lake, blaring AC/DC music through the car, just like they did in the weight room for football lifting.

Having just been at a demolition derby, they sped down the roads, took sharp turns, and slammed the brakes on the way to the lake. The boys were on a high that was about to become a drastic low. They parked at the lake where some friends remained, drinking by the bonfire, and it was quiet. When they turned off the ignition and got out of the car, all they could hear was screaming and banging noises. The girls had been in the trunk for about three hours at that point, and the aggressive driving had led to their injuries.

Samantha said, "Well, you can't make this shit up! And that's why I'm not having kids!"

Fortunately, the girls survived. Eventually they went to rehab centers for physical and occupational therapy and then returned home. The fathers pressed charges, and needless to say, the girls broke up with their boyfriends.

CHAPTER 22
Doctor Google

The interns agreed that "knowledge is power" and that "information can be empowering." However, misinformation can lead to a lot of problems. Our society currently has good and bad information at its fingertips. Within a few seconds anyone can look up information about any subject they desire, including healthcare. During the intern year, Robert, David, and Samantha always told patients, "Be careful with Dr. Google—three clicks and you'll be dying."

These searches do cause a lot of anxiety. During emergency department rotations, each intern saw patients come in for nonsense reasons, telling the interns they looked it up online where they read it could be an emergency. They may see a new bump or lump, or have a new pain, or hear about a new illness, and this leads them down the anxiety-fueled path of Internet searches. So yes, hypochondria is on the rise.

No one knew this better than Samantha, who was on the orthopedic trauma service for a couple months. Because the hospital was a metro-area Level 1 trauma center, patients came from hours away by ambulance and helicopter. Some of the most gruesome injuries are taken care of in the trauma bay and operating rooms of this hospital.

The emergency department called the ortho trauma intern on call, and Samantha came speeding down the hall to the trauma bay, smelling cheap alcohol (not the kind on someone's breath, but the kind that comes from burps, farts, and vomiting). She turned past the curtain and saw a screaming young man wearing a local college T-shirt. His arm was clearly dislocated, swollen, and discolored. The patient, vomiting and shaking, was about to pass out from the pain. The personnel were just watching this young college student who wanted to sit up and get pressure off his shoulder and arm. He was also having neck pain.

Samantha noticed something that the others didn't, and it alarmed her. Although the arm was swollen, the hand was starting to turn grey and discolored—not to mention it was cold and the patient had little control over it. There are some cardinal movements for each joint that indicate whether the nerves and muscles are functioning appropriately. In this case there was limited to no motion and no sensation. This was an ischemic limb secondary to trauma. She asked the nurse to page the vascular surgery intern on call, which was Robert. He came down from the vascular lab and joined Samantha.

The patient would not tell anyone what happened. The assumption was he got the arm caught in something, perhaps some sort of machinery, or that he had taken a direct hit. The injury was too isolated to the arm to have been a fight, a motor-vehicle injury, or any other high-impact injury.

Samantha and Robert knew an injury like this typically occurs only with polytrauma; it is not usually isolated. They had only seen this kind of injury with motor-vehicle accidents, machinery accidents, and falls from trees or roofs. The attending physicians were called, and X-rays and CT scans were done quickly, showing a shattered proximal humerus and clavicle. Essentially the shoulder girdle was ripped apart, and the shoulder bones were dusted in numerous pieces. This was no longer a closed arm fracture; this was a situation where this patient's arm would likely need to be amputated quickly.

The patient's panicked parents arrived and were let into the trauma bay. They had just driven down on a Friday night from a city north of the hospital and, according to the father, had made a 60-mile drive in 35 minutes. It was now 3:00 a.m., and the college student continued to refuse to tell his parents and the healthcare team what happened.

Talking to the parents, Robert said, "Well, it looks like a gorilla yanked his arm tonight." He smiled at the patient, who was now doped up on IV opioids. The surgery team had obtained consent and were ready to go back. Robert walked beside his hospital bed as it was wheeled to the operating room, then the patient went in to be prepared by the anesthesia and surgery teams.

At the scrub sink, Robert stood beside Samantha, shaking his head and looking off in the distance.

Samantha said, "What's wrong with you?" She thought that he was worried about a 19-year-old losing his arm during the surgery. A limb can be without blood flow for only so much time before necrosis and gangrene start. The plans were for orthopedics to attempt to fix an open reduction, internal fixation fracture, and for the vascular team to do a live angiogram to see where the blood flow was blocked and whether bone reduction could restart perfusion. If not, vascular surgery would plan for a bypass. This was going to be at best a six-hour endeavor, but it could go on the whole next day. Even if they were successful, there was a high probability the patient would end up with an amputation in the near future.

Robert told Samantha he wasn't tired, even though it was three in the morning; he was just in disbelief, as were the young man's parents. He told her the story the patient had finally revealed.

The patient was drunk at the local college frat house. They were playing Edward Forty Hands, which Robert admitted he'd played many times before. (This is a game where players typically duct-tape a 40-ounce can of malt liquor to each hand. The participants race to see who can drink the full 80 ounces the quickest. It's a brutal college tradition, especially if—like this patient—you're not an alcoholic. Not only do you get intoxicated quickly, but most people end up urinating on themselves because they can't use their hands with 40-ounce bottles of alcohol taped to them—they can't undo a zipper. Most people have an extended bladder and can't control the urge. You drink all the malt liquor and then others remove the bottles from your hands.)

During this party, while his hands were duct-taped, people started being loud and obnoxious (hard to imagine with that much alcohol consumption).

"Was it Colt 45?" Samantha interrupted. Robert replied, "How would I know?" (It turned out Samantha was a Billie D. Williams fan and loved that old malt liquor commercial.)

So, while all the young men were jumping up and running around, this patient decided to chest bump his best friend. When this happened, he fell backwards with his arm behind him.

Samantha said, "No way. What a freak accident! It's not possible that caused this injury." Robert replied, "No, that's how he dislocated his shoulder. It has nothing to do with this injury."

Robert went on to tell her that once the shoulder was dislocated with a closed fracture, the party came to a halt as the patient screamed in pain and ran around. The 40-ounce drinks, which had spilled everywhere and were warm by then, were removed from his hands. No one knew what to do, and they were afraid to call the authorities because they thought they would be charged with underage drinking and other fines. (All too often this fear leads to injuries and deaths on college campuses. Check the news at the start of the college year and in the late summer and early fall; numerous students throughout the country are injured or die when they could have gotten help.)

One of the frat brothers was in his first year of pre-med studies, and he had an idea. The group decided to google "shoulder dislocation" and then watched numerous YouTube videos on how to relocate the shoulder. The problem was the dislocation was atypical in the pattern of the arm to the shoulder girdle (meaning the shoulder went anterior and distal, to be specific). The videos they watched weren't going to work, but they didn't know that. First, they had the patient put his arm over a chair and one of the stronger frat brothers pulled at the wrist. This only made the patient scream in pain and grab his shoulder.

"You won't believe what this drunk group of shit-for-brains did next, Samantha!" said Robert. "What?" Samantha said, finishing up scrubbing her hands before walking with Robert into the operating room.

Since yanking the arm didn't work, they decided they needed more force, Robert continued, but they couldn't figure out how to get more force. Initially they thought about dropping something off the upstairs balcony that weighed a lot and yanking the arm further, which was just going to make the injury worse. Thankfully they didn't do this, as the patient probably would have gotten a head injury from falling over the balcony to the first floor.

So, these drunk young college students came up with a more effective plan. Although they hadn't gotten this idea from YouTube, they thought surely this would work, and luckily one of them had a pickup truck. They tied a rope to his shoulder and then to a trailer hitch.

Samantha said, "You've got to be kidding me! How is his arm still attached?"

The students helped hold the patient still and slowly the driver moved the truck forward. Fortunately, before the arm was pulled off or disarticulated at the shoulder, someone at the house next door called 911. The patient's pattern of injury was one of the most difficult the 34-year veteran orthopedic trauma surgeon—who had operated in Vietnam—had ever seen. If the good Samaritan hadn't called 911, it was hard to tell what these drunk college students would have tried next. Perhaps the patient was lucky his arm was shattered, that he had no other injuries, and that he lived through this incident.

Nine months later, and after numerous surgeries, the patient still hadn't recovered. The arm was saved, but he will have lifelong chronic pain and swelling with little function of the extremity, a life-changing situation for this young man.

After the fracture was reduced and pinned, and prior to his return for revisional surgery with plate, screws, and a cadaver bone graft, the blood flow was returned. Unfortunately, this resulted in reperfusion syndrome, which is adding blood to an area without blood that leads to compartment syndrome, where the blood goes into an area of the body too rapidly and puts pressure on the nerves, muscles, and soft tissue. This is a surgical emergency and commonly leads to kidney failure. After opening the compartments, the patient eventually required skin grafting from plastic surgery.

At a young age he went to a rehabilitation facility to learn to use his other hand. He is no longer in college, and his friendships at the frat house are ruined as the driver of the truck and others were arrested. A civil case is pending regarding paying medical bills and compensating him for his pain and suffering. After all, it's the American way!

CHAPTER 23
Numb Numb Numb

Robert was the first on surgery rotations and assigned to plastic surgery. What people often don't understand is at a Level 1 trauma center, plastic surgery is more Civil War surgery and less cosmetic surgery. If someone has a burn, a mangled limb, a facial abscess, or needs amputation, etc., the plastics team is called in to perform surgery. (There is a required fellowship for breast surgery, and that is a whole different world. Typically, those are performed by either a cancer or cosmetic surgeon; either way, it's different from plastic reconstructive surgery.)

The attending was Dr. Wilson, and he invented the term "old school." He walked as if he had Parkinson's and was slow and mean with every step. However, when he was under the lights of the operating room, he was fast, efficient, and truly magical to watch—a master of his craft. He had been a surgeon during the Vietnam War and was cool under pressure.

Throughout the surgical day, Robert endured a beating from Dr. Wilson. He seemed to do everything wrong He was anxious but did not let it show, much like an athlete would.

In the next-to-last case, the patient had previously had a CABG (coronary artery bypass graft) and had a host of medical problems. The incision had opened on his chest and caused a wound, for which the patient had a wound vac, a suction device designed with tubing to pull in healthy tissue and decrease drainage.

The plan was for Dr. Wilson and Robert to take the omentum (a mesh-like covering over the intestines) and flip it upside down to cover the heart and structures around it in preparation for grafting to this site. This is not only high risk and intense, it's also a long surgery, taking about seven hours. Part of the reason it took this long, though, was Robert's fault.

He retracted the tissue and asked for the wrong instrument—a sharp instrument that was supposed to be dull. When he gave it to Dr. Wilson, he thought it was the correct, dull instrument, and unfortunately it pierced the heart.

The cardiothoracic surgeon on call was brought in, and he was upset. To Robert, it seemed every other word was a curse word. He had to remain scrubbed and help although he wanted to run away and hide. *Go on to the next play*, he thought, referencing his football experiences. *Don't let this one stop you*. The CT surgeon repaired the heart, and the surgery was completed.

After the case, Robert realized he had sweated through his entire scrubs. He went to change, and there was one more case: a breast reduction. Typically, this case would not worry him, but after his recent mistake, he was nervous.

Thankfully the anesthesia team switched, and Dr. Perry was the anesthesiologist. He was known as one of the funniest attendings at the hospital and was able to keep things light. Robert was not very experienced and looked forward to the distraction.

The surgery was on a 20-year-old, beautiful, voluptuous woman. Looking at her on the operating room table, not only did Robert understand why her back hurt, but he also wondered how she could keep from falling forward when she walked. Likely due to a hormonal issue, her breasts were larger than most porn stars. She wanted a reduction, and everyone agreed this was the right choice. The question was, however, how they were going to make a GGG into a C cup without much scarring, given the redundant skin.

Before the surgery, the patient said that it didn't matter what it looked like, as long as the size was reduced. However, everyone knew that she was concerned about aesthetics. This was a 20-year-old college student, a knockout, who likely had been hounded by boys her age (and men) since she was a teenager because of her large breasts. It's a sad reality she was objectified even before adulthood and what led to this now is the source of significant daily back pain.

Robert walked to the operating table to set up and asked for the local anesthesia, an injection much like you get at the dentist office to numb an area of your mouth. Even though they were using anesthesia, less is used if the area is numb and the patient is asleep.

Next, Dr. Perry piped up from the head of the bed, "Hey, Robert, mind if I help numb the breast?" Then he motioned his head rapidly back and forth, making an eating and nibbling movement with his mouth, saying, "Numb numb numb numb," acting like he was eating the breast.

Robert burst out in laughter. It was a 10-second encounter that made his day. He felt like he was back home and could joke and see the bigger picture. He quickly realized what all seasoned surgeons and anesthesiology doctors know: the operating room is high risk and humor is required for anyone to handle such high-stress levels.

In the medical community, we are saddened by the recordings of doctors that have been viewed in our politically correct culture as inappropriate. Many times, no malice is intended; they are just trying to break the ice in the operating room. In studies, surgeons are shown to perform better when they are relaxed.

That's exactly what happened to Robert. He relaxed and did a great job because of one simple joke. The patient was not aware and would not remember. Perhaps the nurses in the room were offended, perhaps not. The operating room nurses are the toughest of the bunch, can joke around with anyone, and typically are not fazed by much.

Many of you reading this book joke around at work and don't take things too seriously. Well, we have to take things seriously, and we must find a way to lighten the tension. After all, another mistake like Robert made earlier could not only kill the career of a future successful surgeon, but it could also kill a patient and affect families' lives.

As Robert exited the operating room, en route to table rounds (during which attendings and residents typically sit in a circle and go over patients on computers and written notes), he heard the anesthesiologist say, "Hey, young doc, I know you were slow today, but remember there's only one thing you do quickly the first time in life. Everything else takes time to become more efficient."

Robert burst out laughing again like a young adolescent hearing his first sex joke!

CHAPTER 24
Whoopsie

Samantha was assigned to a palliative care rotation run by multiple physicians that were the leaders of a sought-after fellowship program. However, it was known throughout the hospital that the service wasn't run by the attending physicians, fellows, or residents. It was run by a nurse practitioner who had done palliative care for over 45 years and who had been a nurse for 52 years. She was "old school" and stern; she had trained with nurses who started when they were 18 years old and wore the white dress and cap. Her name was Evelyn, and she had the prettiest smile and loudest laugh—you could hear it from down the hallway.

Evelyn had a great outlook on life and was strong in her faith. A devoted Catholic, she told everyone about it, which clashed with the administration who thought her end-of-life "Christian propaganda" hadn't kept up with the times. Additionally, the hospital services a large Muslim population, and her religious views didn't always go over well. It had been known for a few years that Evelyn was showing signs of dementia, and this was starting to impact her job.

Samantha had heard all of this from the last intern who was on the service, but she was looking forward to a break from surgery, which entailed long hours and was high pressure, and moving to a more routine schedule that was internal-medicine based. This routine schedule meant she got to eat lunch every day on the rotation with Evelyn and her team of palliative care nurses.

She was concerned about dealing with a 70-plus-year-old early dementia nurse practitioner in charge of her rotation. Was this a safe situation for the hospital? Maybe, maybe not. Administration can't always keep ahead of these issues, and by the end of our intern year, Evelyn was unfortunately asked to retire, which she did but not without a lengthy legal fight. See, after high school, she went to nursing school at our hospital and had stayed on for work. Her whole life was dedicated to working for the hospital.

After giving them over 50 years of service, it was hard for Evelyn to swallow when they turned on her—as it would be for anyone. I heard she moved to St. Thomas and is living a great life. It turned out she really enjoyed the work; it wasn't about the money. Her husband was a retired international businessman, which explained how she could take these great weekend trips and not miss work. For example, when Samantha was on, she finished with Evelyn at 6:00 p.m. on a Friday and met with her at 6:30 a.m. on Monday to discuss patients. Evelyn asked Samantha how her weekend went, and she told Evelyn she was on call house officer and it was a nightmare. Evelyn told her that was too bad as she had spent the weekend in Costa Rica! Samantha said that was great and talked to her about it, thinking she was just demented. In reality, she had gone to Costa Rica on a private plane her husband owned.

While Samantha was on the rotation, she was both amused and enamored by the way Evelyn would question her patients in the room on rounds and even on phone calls when she followed up with palliative care patients after they left the hospital and were on hospice at home. Evelyn, who obviously had some hearing loss as well, would yell in the phone or room, "Have you pooped today?!" and the patient would answer. With every patient encounter and call, this was the main question, and it blew Samantha's 27-year-old mind until one of the fellows on the service explained that elderly patients get focused on their bowel movements and get upset if they're not regular—particularly if they're constipated for a couple days and are uncomfortable and in pain.

Samantha thought to herself, *I'm a surgery intern, and I can't even tell you the last time I had a bowel movement.* When Samantha was originally on house officer, the senior resident running the service was a power-hungry woman from a white-collar family who had been to the best undergraduate and medical school and wasn't going to be talked down to. She was now the senior in charge—where she belonged—and everyone was going to be subservient to her. This senior resident would not let Samantha go to the bathroom while on the house officer rotation, a situation that ended when Samantha was hospitalized for a bladder and kidney infection and had to take an antibiotic for the next six months. After all that she couldn't understand how holding a bowel movement for more than a day could be of the upmost importance.

Unfortunately, Samantha was on the palliative care service when Evelyn lost it and affected the hospital and patient care. Dealing with dying patients all day as they realize their urgent mortality and lack of time left is a stressful job and difficult on its own. However, when you add in the family, who is often stressed and blames the hospital or staff for their family member's decline, this becomes a volatile situation.

In the mornings Evelyn again was antiquated in her patient care, printing off the patient list and rounding on all of them. Then she would chart-check, write notes, and follow up with all the patients again. She had a new patient list and an established patient list on the electronic medical record system, but she admitted she preferred paper charts and wasn't good at the computer.

On this day with Samantha, who waited for Evelyn to print lists as usual and then proceed to rounding, there were 32 patients on the established patient list and 21 on the new patient list, which Samantha thought was unusually high.

Evelyn looked at it and said, "Okay, we've got a lot of new consults and need to get going. Gravity rounds," she reported, which meant they would start at the top floor rounding and take the stairs until all the floors with patients were seen and they were at the bottom floor of patients. Samantha went with Evelyn, noting the fellow was off this day for a conference, and started rounds on the top floor of the hospital.

Each time they went into a patient room, Samantha did a quick exam of the heart, lungs, and extremities while Evelyn talked to the patients. Evelyn was masterful in the way she broke the news to a patient that they were terminally ill, probably due in part to the fact that she had done it thousands of times. The patients typically expected the news, at least somewhat, but were still in an element of shock hearing it for the first time officially and taking in the information. After a great discussion, she would then go into direct, brash questions such as, "Have you pooped today?!"

This day on rounds, though, the patients weren't stoic and shocked—they were downright flabbergasted and confused. They seemed angry and upset, saying things like, "How could this be?!" over and over, patient after patient. The patients also didn't fit the normal demographic. Samantha noticed patients in their 20s and 30s that appeared otherwise healthy. After seeing the 15th patient, Samantha realized the physical exams she was doing while Evelyn talked to the patients were similar. All the patients were in casts or splints to their extremities; some were even in neck collars and traction.

After the 16th patient, Samantha got up the nerve to say something to Evelyn, not expecting it to go well. How could a 20-something female question a professional 70-something female in the workplace? Well, medical staff are empowered to speak up if they see something wrong and cannot be punished for reporting in good faith.

Samantha said to Evelyn, "Are you sure these are the correct patients? They're all so taken aback by the news that they're dying, and they seem younger than most of our patients."

"I've run this service since you were in diapers," Evelyn replied. "I know what I'm doing. Disease doesn't discriminate" She went on to explain that age, gender, race, color, socioeconomic status, etc. don't matter with terminal diseases. "If you can't handle it, perhaps you're not cut out to be a physician after all," Evelyn added.

Shocked and shut down, Samantha simply said, "Okay," and kept following Evelyn. Although she had been cut down much worse in the operating room, this was different. She knew something was wrong.

Samantha's residency program director was known for asking residents, "Are you stupid, or do you just not care? You've got to be one of those to have made such a terrible patient care mistake." As a consequence, Samantha spent many hours in an operating room thinking that not only had she made a mistake that could have been devastating to patient care and their families, she also wondered, *Which am I? Lazy, uncaring, or stupid?* Thinking about that a lot can drive some residents to the brink. Surgery residents typically develop Stockholm syndrome, in which hostages or abuse victims bond with their captors or abusers until the abuse becomes normal to them and they feel unsettled without the abuse. Ask any surgeon about this, and they'll tell you it's exactly how they learned in training.

Samantha and Evelyn saw the final five patients, and now on the bottom patient floor, they headed to the physicians' room for documentation. Samantha hadn't said more than a peep since Evelyn cut her down. As Evelyn sat down to document and chart, Samantha got ready to tell her about her physical exam findings when she looked down at the rounding list. The established patient list of 32 patients said "Palliative Care" on the top, and the new patient list of 21 patients said "Ortho Surg" on the top.

"You've got to be kidding me," Samantha said. "Evelyn, look at these lists!" Samantha pointed to the top of the patient list. It was a simple mistake. The orthopedic service list had been left in the printer, and Evelyn grabbed the top two pieces of paper from the printer without looking at them. One was the established palliative care list and the other the orthopedics rounding list. Evelyn simply hadn't taken the time to look.

"This can't be correct!" Evelyn yelled and started to stomp around angrily.

All the physicians were looking at them. Samantha didn't realize Evelyn was on a short leash with administration because of the early dementia signs against which she had adamantly fought, saying people didn't like her and were trying to get rid of her. Samantha couldn't wrap her head around what had happened that morning, and Evelyn couldn't bring herself to admit that she had told 21 orthopedic patients that were admitted for fractures and other traumas or infections that they were going to die in the near future. No wonder the patients looked perplexed and angry; they were otherwise healthy and told incorrectly that they were terminal.

Everyone knows it's best to admit fault in the healthcare system and not cover it up. Patients are smarter than you think, and providers need to admit to any mistakes immediately. Evelyn had Samantha come with her to help cover her tracks. She was ready to admit the mistakes, but she was too late. In each patient room there were either family members present or family members on the phone—there was even a pastor bedside.

Evelyn did her best to explain what happened, but no one understood. "How could this be?" they asked. The patients were on a roller coaster of emotions: one minute they were dying and the next they were fine and being discharged that day.

On top of all that, as luck would go, that day the attending running the orthopedic service (known for being an arrogant bunch of attending surgeons at our hospital) was the most arrogant of them all. He was livid and calling for Evelyn's and Samantha's heads.

Samantha was eventually reprimanded but forgiven by the medical education department and continued her residency—though with many ugly, unfortunate meetings. The patients all lived (as far as we know), and the hospital system ended up writing off their bills—likely to keep it from making it to the local and national news stations. Shortly thereafter Evelyn was relieved of her position. If she had just done the new-age chart-checking prior to rounding, this could have easily been avoided. The old surgery and carpentry saying applies in all situations: "Measure twice and cut once."

CHAPTER 25
Bizarre Patients, Bizarre Doctors

Thanks to the combination of being overworked and stressed, the eccentric personalities of attending physicians, and literally insane patients, intern year blurs the lines between being in the real world, make believe, and being in a dream state. The interns learned that repetition and study under duress can make a great physician and surgeon who becomes objective and robotic. The problem lies outside the hospital with relationships with others who have not had this experience, and the overwhelming stress that comes from the intern year. All the interns' relationships at home and with family started to sour as they were viewed as cynical, quick-tempered, and fatigued.

Samantha drove her car into a median on the interstate when she fell asleep at the wheel after a house officer shift. David flew to a conference, fell asleep in the aisle seat far before the three-hour trip started, and only woke up when the stewardess started slapping him on the chest. He had slept through the flight, the landing, two other passengers going either over or around him, and everyone else leaving the plane. Robert fell asleep while walking in his neighborhood and apparently landed in a neighbor's front yard before coming to. In other words, work was tiring!

Robert was on service with a seasoned surgeon who was excellent when it came to the technical aspects and medical decisions, but whose bedside manner was a nightmare. Despite Robert's efforts to try to coach the attending on rounds when presenting, telling him the patient was foreign or of foreign ancestry but spoke English well, the attending would mess it up. For instance, Robert told the attending that the patient was Hispanic but had been born and raised here. What did the attending do? He yelled at the patient, speaking English slowly the entire time. Robert shook his head and thought to himself, *Hey, dumbass, the patient is Hispanic not deaf.*

In another incident at the end of a case with a deaf patient who read lips very well, the patient started fighting with the operating room staff as he came out of anesthesia. This can be dangerous; when patients wake up from anesthesia and don't know where they are, they sometimes start violently fighting the staff and their restraints. If they aren't controlled, patients can pull out their IV access lines and injure themselves—even scratching their eyes, resulting in corneal damage. Some patients come out of anesthesia early and try to pull out their own airways. There is amnesia medication for this, so the patient doesn't usually remember these events. When this deaf, violent patient came to, the oblivious attending surgeon got in front of his face and started yelling at the patient, calling him by his name and telling him to calm down.

The patient kept fighting, however, and the attending kept yelling, telling the staff, "It's okay—the patient can read lips." No one wanted to say anything to this powerful, awkward attending about a problem getting in the way of the patient's understanding.

Robert contemplated the situation for a bit, then while holding the patient down, he said to the attending, "He reads lips and you're still wearing a mask!"

Robert took a tongue-lashing after embarrassing the attending in front of the operating room staff and anesthesia team, but they all had a good laugh about it later behind the attending's back. When the mask was removed, the patient did understand he was in an operating room and calmed right down.

Later that day Robert and the attending headed to the emergency department to see a patient who was (by all accounts) insane and needed to be in the psychiatric ward. However, he had been stabbed in a street fight. The patient had internal bleeding and had actually been found to have a gunshot wound to his leg as well. The patient needed surgery, and Robert prepared to get consent and to get the operating room ready. Because it's rare to have both gunshot and knife wounds, Robert questioned the patient with the attending.

The patient had been wanted by the police for quite some time, and the police were outside the room; the patient was now in custody. Apparently, the patient had become somewhat of a vigilante over the past month in the inner city, shooting and killing people, providing his own justice instead of calling the police. There had been manhunts for the patient for months, but he could not be found. Whenever he killed someone in a certain neighborhood (whether it was true vigilantism or serial killing is not known), he would put a large Batman sticker on a nearby stop sign or building sign. It was a bizarre crime ritual.

The patient also had a Batman tattoo on his face, though he seemed normal and was very engaging and charismatic in conversation. Robert almost found himself forgetting all the murders the patient had committed. (This is common with psychotics; studies show their heart rate doesn't go up in high-stress situations and that they can be calming and dominant in conversations. The patient would be in a psychiatric ward or jail hopefully for the remainder of his life.) Robert couldn't get past staring at the patient's Batman tattoo on his face and neither could the staff or the attending.

After getting the consent signed, Robert was walking out of the patient's room with the attending, headed to the elevator to go to the operating room, when the attending turned to Robert and said, "Well, I guess someone else will have to clean up the streets of Gotham now!"

CHAPTER 26
Confidence, Not Arrogance

It was toward the end of the intern year, and Samantha, David, and Robert were about to be residents (or PGY-2 status, which means post-graduate from medical school, second-year residents), which comes with less time on the house officer rotation.

Students were still doing audition months, meaning fourth-year medical students were spending a month in different hospitals and then interviewing to hopefully match or receive a job offer as a resident with the hospital. This month there was an intelligent, arrogant male student from a wealthy American family, the kind of person who had never been told no, whose parents told him every day he was better than everyone. He walked with the sense of entitlement that drove the interns insane. Samantha was the daughter of two factory workers, and she was smarter and more experienced than this student, and she knew it. The problem with this kind of young male is that they many times don't respect females, particularly ones with power.

Samantha got a call from the emergency department about a frequent flyer (a patient who commonly came into the emergency department not for an actual issue but for laughs with the staff and physicians to see what he could get away with) on their service. The patient was a unique, mid-30s male with a unilateral arthrogryposis of his left arm. Arthrogryposis is a connective-tissue neuromuscular disorder in which there can be multiple contractures of joints since birth. It is studied in medical school and seen in some children, though it's rare in children, even rarer in adults, and exceedingly rare for it to be unilateral as many times it affects all joints.

"What is his presenting complaint this time?" Samantha asked the emergency room doctor.

"Broken wrist, of course!" the ER doctor responded.

Samantha was about to round up the students to see the patient when she had an idea. She called the arrogant medical student and asked him to see the patient in emergency department room 52.

"It's an arm fracture," Samantha told him. "I know you want to get into orthopedics, so this should be right up your alley. If it's displaced, go ahead and reduce it, then we'll come down and get post-reduction X-rays. Thanks for the help."

Samantha went to the physicians' bay in the emergency department, right around the corner from the patient's room where she could eavesdrop on the patient encounter. The student didn't even introduce himself; he just started talking brashly to the man, telling him about the fracture and what he was going to do. The patient, who obviously had a psychological problem, was really into it. (Remember, he was just doing this to mess with staff. Sometimes he got imaging, including CT scans and other diagnostics, and if he was lucky, he got to mess with an intern or two. Today was his lucky day to pull one over on an arrogant student.) Samantha really enjoyed this and thought it would be a great learning experience in life lessons and humility.

The patient told an elaborate story about a slip-and-fall injury while climbing a mountain in another country, and the student wasn't even listening to him. He said he suffered the injury and flew back here by private plane just to have the student help him, pretending to be so grateful.

The student missed several clues, and as a fourth-year medical student, he should have been more aware; however, arrogance and lack of experience led him down this path. Medical students across the country have to do observed patient encounters with actors who are paid to present different complaints. Many schools throughout the United States send their students to the Philadelphia area to do this live mock exam for pass/fail, and others do these individually at their school or at a nearby training location. Plus, the student had an entire year or more of patient care, so he should have been able to calm down and see what was in front of him.

The student struggled mightily, and fortunately for the patient, he had neuropathy from advanced alcoholism. Samantha let him struggle until she'd had enough. She fiercely pulled back the curtain and looked into the student's eyes. He was shaking and mumbled something about not being able to reduce the fracture.

Samantha said, "Did you even look at the X-rays closely? Didn't you ever study in school about arthrogryposis?"

The student simply put his head down and turned bright red while Samantha and the patient laughed.

It's unbelievable that the patient continues to make it past nursing triage. If they would just look at his notes, they'd catch him. However, when they see the deformed arm and hear the patient's convincing story, they immediately jump to rooming him in the emergency department. Samantha had seen the patient many times before, and this wouldn't be the last time either. She enjoyed the "learning experience" the student had, and he started respecting her and doing what she said, probably because he didn't want her to tell others about this incident.

Shaking her head, Samantha asked the student, "What's more disturbing and dangerous—a medical student who's arrogant who becomes a doctor who thinks he knows it all and hurts patients, or a psychotic alcoholic who thinks it's fun to spend his free time in emergency departments?" She paused, then said, "The dangerous doctor for sure, as he can affect more people." Samantha went on to explain to the medical student, "Honesty is always best, particularly in the surgery world. We're all human and make mistakes. You will never know how far a genuine, sincere 'I'm sorry' or 'I don't know the answer, but I'll find out' can go with patients."

CHAPTER 27
It's Going Tibia Okay

One problem with the intern year is that the older residents typically stick the med students on the interns to manage. This is inappropriate because the intern is often drowning under their workload, and having to manage (and keep an eye on) someone who knows less than them is a daunting task. The more seasoned residents should monitor and educate the medical students; the interns don't have time to teach. As one now-retired surgery attending used to say, "You spend the intern year at the hospital just trying to figure out where the bathroom is!"

The medical students came from schools throughout the country and grew up in many different states and cultures and had many different accents and mannerisms. During the intern year at Robert, David, and Samantha's teaching hospital—considered one of the best in the region and perhaps one of the top in the country—there was a host of bad medical students.

A large number of these students had a poor work ethic, they were book smart but not street smart, and they were entitled. Initially these problems were blamed on the fact that they were part of the millennial generation, which has taken the brunt of jokes and blame in the media as well as in other careers. However, some of the millennials were fantastic, highly motivated, smart individuals. The interns couldn't put their finger on the reason why it was an off year, but it was a scary harbinger for future generations of residents.

The following is an anecdote featuring one of these students: One of the hospital's pleasant, laid-back attendings was running rounds with a group of fellows, residents, interns, and students. (This is essentially what you see on TV or in the movies when one head doctor is followed by up to 10 other doctors—you know, the part where patients get intimidated and don't remember who's in their room.) This attending liked non-fellows and residents to stay outside in the hallway as he did his rounds so as to not overwhelm the patient with a large number of people. When this attending, who was normally reserved and quiet, came out of the room and saw one of the students was on his iPad, he ignored it and continued rounds. The student continued on his iPad until the attending made an unusual request that the student come into the next post-operative patient's room with the others, instead of staying in the hall. The student already had his PhD and was awaiting his MD, and he appeared annoyed by this opportunity.

As the intern, Robert was in the hallway with the other students and a resident who had stayed behind when he heard, "What the fuck is your problem?" Robert's mouth fell open. The attending had a deep, dooming voice, and Robert had never even heard him say anything bad about anyone over the course of the year, let alone yell at anyone.

The attending came blazing out of the room with everyone else in tow, including the student, who looked white as a ghost and was putting up his iPad.

As the attending went by, he said, "That shit-for-brains student is checking his stock accounts instead of learning! Send him home!"

So there went the student, kicked out by the senior resident to the "library rotation," meaning he was asked to go to the library and make endless PowerPoints on topics sent by the residents to be quizzed on later.

Another time David was in surgery with a student who was first in their class and came highly recommended, based on their academics—which may have been through the roof, but practical intelligence is another matter. Every year residents take personality tests to pair them with attending physicians, and it wasn't clear what attending this student could be paired with if he joined our program. The student said he had life figured out; his grandparent had died and left him several million dollars. He was distracted and spent more time chasing the female nurses and staff than learning.

David said, "Hey, do you know how to put your gloves on the sterile field [the operating room table]?"

The student scoffed and said, "Of course I know how to put my gloves out. I got this, don't worry."

David went to scrub his hands and heard a loud commotion. He walked in the operating room, and the surgical tech was beside herself. It was right before a stressful case, everything was already set up, and the student grabbed a packet of size 7 gloves from the shelf in the operating room and simply threw the gloves and the packaging on the table, contaminating everything. It all had to be thrown away and redone, and all the instruments had to be sterilized again. This kind of mistake can cost several thousand dollars.

The student was nervous and did show remorse, so David tried to calm him down. The student was a southern gentleman with a thick accent and flowing dark hair. David thought he had seen this guy many times before; you know the type—Croakies sunglass, the straps hanging; a collared shirt with the front tucked into belted short-shorts; and Sperry topsiders. They're too cool for anyone else, but when they're smacked in the face with a problem, they come unglued and can't get it back together. The student was hyperventilating. He was about to scrub into a brain surgery and needed to calm himself.

David said, "Look, you should take a break and sit this case out. Perhaps go to the lounge and eat and drink something. Maybe your blood glucose is low, and you're not thinking right." The student was adamant. He wanted to stay and eventually be part of the residency program.

David said, "Look, this is your first brain surgery. If you feel like you're going to pass out, just sit down—and bend your knees ahead of time—and just sit on the floor. The staff will help you. It's easy to watch something in lecture halls and on YouTube; however, when it's real and happening in front of you, it's not for the faint of heart."

About midway through the case, David noticed the student making some strange sounds under his mask. David couldn't tell what was going on, and the student looked wide-eyed and afraid. David thought the student was probably panicking because the attending surgeon was so quiet and intimidating. Then the attending noticed and asked if the student was okay. He didn't say anything; he just nodded his head up and down, indicating "yes."

By this time the student's cheeks were obviously engorged, and he was pulling on his mask. Sweat was coming through his cap. The next thing David knew, the student had vomited in his mask, though he initially refused to walk away until the nursing staff made him as he was no longer sterile. He was willing to continue on regardless of being sick and endangering others. At least he was committed!

Robert may have had the worst student of all. The student was a hairy, overweight gentlemen of Greek background who was funny and had a great personality; his interpersonal skills were sure to make up for his lack of common sense and book smarts. The student was asked to not be involved directly with the surgery and only observe from a distance.

He was to step back and observe a trauma case. (In other words, the other physicians didn't want him in the way but still wanted to provide a learning experience.) The student squeezed into scrubs that were too small for him, and his chest hair and the gold chain around his neck really stood out. He was crowding the surgeon and residents who asked him many times to step back. (Imagine operating on someone with a blade in your hand and literally feeling someone breathing on the back of your neck.)

Well, he didn't listen; he didn't back up during an open abdominal exploration surgery. As luck would have it, a large hematoma under pressure came flying off the surgical field and over the attending's shoulder, who moved slightly to avoid it and continued to work. The hematoma was the size of half a head of lettuce, and it landed square on the student's chest above the scrubs. As the glob of blood that closely resembled currant jelly stuck to his chest hair and started to slowly slide down his abdomen, the student lost consciousness, unfortunately landing directly on the back of his head in the operating room.

Instead of taking him to the trauma bay, imaging was brought to him, and he was taken to surgery emergently by the neurosurgeon for a brain bleed. Robert thought this was fitting to life: one moment you're crowding and pushing your way around, and the next moment you're flat on your back with a brain bleed.

The struggling students were by far at their worst and had poor luck when they weren't being directly supervised. Other memorable issues that occurred during the intern year included the following: Two students were practicing injections on each other with local anesthetics and learning different joint injections. In the lab, one student injected a local anesthetic into what he thought was the anterior shoulder of the other, but it turned out to be the right upper lobe of the other student's lung. Her lung immediately collapsed, and she was rushed to ICU for a chest tube. She lived but missed a month of education, and her parents had to fly in from out of town to care for her.

Another incident involved an unfortunate student who was about to graduate medical school. After a day at the hospital, the student was crossing the city street heading for the parking garage, trusting the crosswalk signs and failing to look. That was when one of the city bus drivers didn't stop—because he was having his first TIA (transient ischemic attack, meaning a "mini stroke"). The bus hit the student and pinned them against the wall; while the student was pinned, the bus driver's foot remained stuck on the gas pedal! The passengers on the bus got the driver's foot off and put the bus in park.

The student went through numerous surgeries and spent approximately six weeks in the hospital—of course, all free of charge, courtesy of the hospital and bus company. There is certainly a lawsuit on the horizon. The student will have to miss at least a year of medical school, and although they're alive, they will live with chronic pain and drastically altered life.

There was no intentional fault here, but lives were changed that day. Around the hospital, people talked about the lawsuit numbers, which are typically based on future earnings. This was a medical student with 50 years of physician's earnings ahead of them! Of course, the real talk should have been if the accident hadn't occurred across the street, the patient would not be alive today. If you're going to have a polytrauma, having it across the street from a Level 1 trauma center is where to do it.

CHAPTER 28
It's Just Business

All physicians (and even the interns) face the reality of healthcare being big business. It is consumer- and administrator-driven, which is in stark contrast to previous generations of physicians who practiced with autonomy. Not only do patients question every decision while googling a diagnosis, but insurance mandates what can and can't be done. More than ever, physicians have to keep patient care first and be an advocate for their patient. Being stripped of making healthcare decisions and being questioned while doing it is one of the driving factors behind physician burnout, substance abuse, and the dramatic increase in suicide rates (add student loan debt, as well as societal expectations and rules, and the rates are worse).

Did you know that physicians in some states are now allowed the privilege of seeing a mental health professional at least one time without being reported to the state medical board? This is a big step in the right direction, but it is not a fix.

Many times, physicians have to hide their mental health struggles and self-medicate, hoping the licensing agency and oversight don't find out, which ultimately hurts the patients. Unfortunately, some physicians are addicted to pain pills and are writing prescriptions for themselves, or they are drunk while seeing patients. Worse yet, they trade pain pill prescriptions and other favors for sex with patients in their office or at other locations.

Another problem is basing patient treatment decisions on money or having to consult with companies or hospitals designed to save healthcare dollars and send money back to physicians and practices. This can lead to aggressive care and skewed decision-making.

Along these lines, Robert was on the phone one day in the resident lounge actively arguing to get an MRI approved with an insurance company. The attending orthopedist didn't want to make the call and "turfed" (dumped) this duty on the intern. Here Robert was, trying to get an approval for an MRI of a patient's ankle, and he was struggling. First, Robert didn't know the patient case well; he was simply looking through the notes the attending's staff sent him to review. He was growing agitated as the other person on the line didn't make any sense and just continued to say, "The answer is no!" The insurance company wasn't going to budge regardless of the argument, and Robert felt disheartened that he couldn't help this patient.

Finally, Robert said, "Sir, can I ask you what your specialty is?" (Many times, the hired physicians at health insurance companies have sold out or couldn't qualify to continue to practice. In the interns' limited experience, they didn't want to become "professional whores"—the physicians who work for insurance companies or are overpaid to testify against physicians as experts, most of whom will say anything to try to win a malpractice suit.)

The doctor on the other end responded, "Optometry."

Robert put his head down on the desk and started to pretend to hit his head with the phone as he said, "I'm calling about an orthopedic ankle MRI and you're an eye doctor!"

Robert thought, *We're speaking two different languages right now*. He had nothing against any eye doctors, be they optometrists or ophthalmologists; what he did have a problem with was a hired doctor who just turned down patient imaging no matter the reason. Robert had hit a roadblock, and the insurance would not cover the imaging. He called the attending who was upset. Apparently, the attending was able to work an al a carte rate with the imaging center, and the patient paid out-of-pocket, likely less than they would have paid as a copay to the insurance company. Again, the doctor without help from the system had to think outside the box for the patient.

Does the United States really want a future where all doctors are stressed about money, student loans, the administration judging their every decision, and not having control of patient care decisions? Who would you rather have to worry about not having enough money to live, the professional athlete or the professional physician who's taking your family member to surgery the next day?

Additionally, we know pediatricians have it the worst financially. Do you want someone caring for your child who is stressed and overwhelmed, thanks to more than $400,000 in student loans (with monthly payments of around $3,000 to the student loan companies), not to mention medical malpractice insurance, DEA fees, state medical and society fees, hospital fees, and so on, while making only $80,000 a year on average?

The current state of healthcare needs an overhaul. The insurance restrictions and the decrease in reimbursements are driving physicians out of private practice and into joining large groups, managed health organizations, or hospitals directly. The interns commonly worried about what the future held.

CHAPTER 29
The Good Ol' Days

Samantha would often hear doctors talk about "the good ol' days of surgery," such as the way the original *M*A*S*H* movie depicted surgeons getting whatever they asked for. The surgeons were the breadwinners (and still are) of the hospital and healthcare system, while the cerebral, likely more intelligent internal medicine physicians and many of their specialties are not reimbursed as much as the proceduralists. Given the mix of older and younger surgeons in the training program, Samantha unfortunately saw the divide and the fight between old-school surgeons and administration.

Samantha thought the goal was to practice autonomously as a physician and never be in the profession so long that the administration tapped on your shoulder and told you that your career was over or—even worse—the state medical board took away your license. The suits from upstairs in administration looked at patients as statistics, and Samantha held nothing against them; it was their job to keep the hospital afloat while managing a host of personalities.

The personalities included the constantly complaining, never-getting-enough older surgeons. Well, during Samantha's intern year, the administration really started to clamp down on the surgeons' requests, setting in motion a process similar to not letting the inmates run the asylum (and yes, the surgeons were the inmates). Many times, a cost-cutting measure would push an attending over the edge and lead to a revolt.

Sometimes meaningless arguments ensued, such as an attending being upset about the type of Gatorade in the surgeon's lounge being changed. Then there were patient-care issues, not having antidote medications to cut costs, changing the process in surgery, and worst of all, limiting the equipment and implants surgeons could use based on hospital saving and reimbursements.

One such event occurred when Samantha was on trauma surgery. One of the heads of trauma was an Australian-born mountain of a man in his mid-60s who was still full of energy and taking 24-hour call shifts. Dr. Taylor had come to America on a football scholarship and played on the practice squad of a famous 1980s NFL team. At six feet, six inches and 235 pounds, he was still in great physical shape with little body fat. He had a well-groomed beard and a Cro-Magnon forehead.

Samantha really enjoyed working with him as he was an incredible surgical teacher. Not only did he keep the room light and fun, he had a way of instructing that made sense for a surgeon in training. When other attendings would get frustrated and not make sense, he would simply tell the interns to turn their hand a certain number of degrees or shift their weight and that would make the case work smoothly.

Samantha happened to be on call the day that the attending retired. He was more than financially ready; he had made a lot of money doing research and held several patents for surgical equipment. He was a well-known name internationally, and he talked to Samantha about the financial pinnacle, where your investments make more money per year than you can earn—a lofty goal for anyone who will remain frugal with their spending.

It was a cold, snowy, windy winter day. Samantha saw the first trauma patient in the morning and had the surgery consents ready. Dr. Taylor came in, signed the forms, and headed to the locker room, where he changed into scrubs, just like any other routine day. Dr. Taylor went into the first operating room and apparently noticed the nurse was wearing a new zip-up cloth cover.

"The new infectious control clothes, I see," said Dr. Taylor. "Do you know you can see your bra and panties through those?" The nurse put her head down in shame, and Dr. Taylor known for his outspoken nature and at times temper started to get angry.

Samantha and Dr. Taylor completed the case (and, frankly, saved the patient's life); however, during the entire case, the doctor kept going on and on about how the suits upstairs had made another asinine decision without consulting the surgeons. Simply put, he was pissed.

As he walked out of the operating room and down the hall, he saw nurses—mostly women but also some men—essentially naked except for their underwear and a see-through infection gown. Dr. Taylor turned to Samantha. "How in the fuck are they getting away with this and no one is saying anything, and how the fuck do they stop the spread of infection if their underwear is exposed?"

"And why don't more nurses wear underwear to work!" Samantha responded, trying to lighten his mood.

It turned out that Dr. Taylor, who had earned the utmost respect of everyone in the hospital even though he could be a hothead, had three daughters—all young professionals who had experienced inappropriate, sexist issues in their respective workplaces. Dr. Taylor however didn't stand for demeaning women and went up to one of the supervisor nurses and asked to speak with her. She agreed to change and gave Dr. Taylor her infection suit.

Then he went to the locker room, and with about 30 minutes to spare before he had to cut on his next patient, Dr. Taylor crammed his six-foot, six-inch, 235-pound frame into a nurse's infection clothes that were meant for someone who weighed no more than 150 pounds. Of course, he took off all his clothes, including his underwear. When he walked by her, Samantha's jaw dropped. You see, he may have been 65 years old, but unknown to everyone, Dr. Taylor was hung like a horse.

Samantha turned to the other interns and said, "What's he got, a pringles can under there?!"

So there went Dr. Taylor, walking out of the surgical area and down the hallway wearing nothing but a millimeter's thickness of see-through cloth in the new infection clothes. He took the public elevator (because why not?), went to the top floor, and walked right into administration. Samantha only heard after the fact, but apparently the secretary was in awe and couldn't speak for a while. Dr Taylor just asked repeatedly to see the president of the hospital. The secretary finally got it together, stopped looking at his crotch, and said the president was busy in a meeting right now with other administrators from the hospital system. She explained he could take a seat and wait or schedule an appointment.

Dr. Taylor said, "Other administrators from the system, huh? Perfect!" And he barged into the conference room.

He walked into the board room, in front of all the hospital presidents in the system, got up on the table, and slowly spun around with his arms up. (You see, when someone is financially secure and tired of the current dogma, they don't care. They just want to get their point across.) Dr. Taylor asked each of them to look at him and asked how stupid could this new policy be? Under the guise of infection control (and also because of laundry costs), the suits didn't allow scrubs to be worn under this.

Dr. Taylor, one of the most prominent trauma surgeons in the country, told the administrators, "Fuck off. I'm retiring when I walk out this door, and you may have a successful hospital again if you put patient care first. There's an idea."

The loss of Dr. Taylor was devastating, and many other attending surgeons left with him, which meant the hospital had to work with locums (for-hire part-time physicians and surgeons) as they slowly started to rebuild the department. Samantha will always reference the legend of Dr. Taylor as a surgeon and the legend of Dr. Taylor's anatomy!

CHAPTER 30
Premiums

Each of the interns—Robert, Samantha, and David—had to cover some outpatient clinic time, which they dreaded. As a Level 1 trauma center, the hospital couldn't turn down patients without insurance, Medicaid, or Affordable Care Act insurance (commonly referred to as Obamacare). While some hospitals have gone to admitting only private-insurance patients and transferring uninsured or Medicaid patients from their emergency departments to this hospital, the Level 1 trauma center is stuck. This can lead to financial tension for the hospital, which wants to make up lost money in the clinics. This means the clinics are typically run by older, angry administrators or nurses who didn't do well in other roles and are stuck on the clinic islands as managers.

The problem with the Affordable Care Act insurance is the patients have an insurance card and can make an appointment, but typically they can't afford to pay their bills or even their copay. However, once they establish legally, they need to be seen. How would you run a business if all or the majority of your services were provided free of charge? This is why you see consolidation with hospital systems and doctors' offices. The private doctor hanging a shingle is quickly going by the wayside.

The interns would laugh when socialized medicine was pushed. In some states, more than 50 percent of the population is on Medicaid; that means the 48 percent of Americans who pay taxes are covering the healthcare costs of those that don't. Even worse, if healthcare were free, would you go to the emergency room or doctor for every little complaint that concerned you, or would you wait until it got so bad you couldn't go on anymore? That's the divide in American healthcare: you have the hardworking Americans who are privately insured through their employer or who purchased insurance on the marketplace who refuse to go to the doctor, follow through with treatments, or follow up because of the cost. They're paying every two weeks out of their checks, they have high deductibles, and they are still paying more.

Even more concerning, if healthcare for all occurs and the government is on the hook financially speaking there will be incentive for the patient to constantly go to the doctors and hospital as its not costing them anything. The hospital in turn is going to be paid no matter what they charge and will quickly raise cost to capitalize on this policy. A slippery slope that could end up with far less physicians in an already short-staffed healthcare system.

David was scheduled to work in the outpatient surgery clinic and was approaching the front entrance around 7:15 a.m. on a Monday when he saw a 40-something, slightly overweight gentlemen bent over, holding his chest. The man's wife was rubbing his shoulders, saying he was going to be okay.

They were leaning on the front door, so when David got close to them, he said, "Can I help you two?"

The wife replied, "He's been having chest pain since yesterday morning and didn't sleep at all last night, but he refused to go to the emergency department because of the cost!" The patient knew one of the nurse practitioners at the clinic and showed up before office hours, waiting for the office to open.

David ushered the man into a room and hooked up the EKG leads. He was in the middle of a NSTEMI, a dangerous heart attack. He was bent over because his body was starving for oxygenated blood.

David called the nurse practitioner the man knew, then the transfer center to admit the patient, and then the cardiologist. Within 45 minutes the patient was in the catheter lab getting his blockage addressed by the cardiologist. David was incredulous that the man would risk his life to avoid the emergency department bill, even with insurance. Unfortunately, this is all too common; ask any physician, and they will tell you a similar story from their practice.

There are those who qualify for Medicaid who—given their below-poverty-line income (on paper)—deserve help as they typically already have risk factors or medical conditions. Sometimes these are obvious physical ailments like a childhood trauma, cancer that left them deformed, MRDD, etc. Sometimes they have a mental health condition, and it's not so readily apparent. However, many patients want to get on disability so that they can get health insurance for free and "get that government money check" as one patient told David in the clinic.

David was covering orthopedics and seeing post-op patients when he saw a patient for right-heel pain. The patient readily admitted she wanted permanent disability from Social Security for plantar fasciitis. David held back his laughter, thinking of all the impaired patients he'd had who couldn't get disability and here sat an overweight 20-something woman with no other medical problems; she just didn't want to work.

There are frustrations with the system. Each intern saw 18-year-old heroin addicts get immediately approved for disability insurance while 60-year-old amputees had to struggle to get their applications reviewed, got denied, had to appeal, and had to involve an attorney or advocacy group to handle their appeal process, which takes a percentage of their back pay. Having Medicaid means free care and no collection agencies if the bills don't get paid. You may not even have to waste gas money to drive as rides are covered. It's a well-designed system for the right reasons, unfortunately it can be exploited. As a self-described southern redneck, David used to get on a soapbox whenever he was asked about this. Unfortunately, early in the year David saw a patient on rounds who complained that their government aid was being decreased to only over $2,000 a month for themselves, their spouse, and a child.

David lost his mind. He was making only $1,500 a month after taxes, had student loans, lived in a tiny apartment, snuck food from the hospital when he was able, and sometimes skipped meals to have more money for his wife and child. David was barely making it and racking up credit cards just to stay afloat while his wife worked also; daycare had been removed from the hospital and was too expensive to afford at the time. He was paying taxes to help this patient get free care who was in no worse shape physically than he was—and he was starving. Of course, his upside was bright, but how much debt would he have piling up at 18 percent interest on his credit cards and over $400,000 in student loans financed at over 7% interest? Somedays David said he should have stopped working and just spent his time tinkering on cars and hunting!

So, if you have Medicaid, the emergency department is free to you, and because of medical malpractice cases, doctors have to practice defensive medicine. The patient goes in with a slight pain on their side; it's likely due to the way they slept or inflammation between the cartilage of the ribs. The patient gets admitted, however, and receives at least a $50,000 workup to rule out cardiac and other reasons for the symptoms. The patient never even sees a bill. Well, as you all know, someone is paying for this—the taxpayer and government.

If this country adopts socialized medicine, perhaps those with insurance and high premiums and deductibles will come in sooner and not suffer in silence, trying to make ends meet for their family as the middle class divides even further. However, tort law would need to be stopped for medical malpractice, and the way physicians practice would need to change. In addition, patients would have to wait for care, which is hard to imagine in this American society where people want something done yesterday.

One of the graduates from the residency program for orthopedics went to Canada to practice and immediately had a booming practice. Apparently in the area where he moved, patients typically waited two to three years for a hip, knee, or ankle replacement. Because he joined a group there, now patients only have to wait about a year and a half for surgery. Imagine experiencing pain with every step you take because of end-stage arthritis in your knee. You've seen a doctor and been told you need a joint replacement.

Everyone in America would say, "Great, let me talk to the surgery scheduler and book it. I can't live like this any longer. Besides, I waited until I could barely walk before coming in to have this looked at."

Imagine then the doctor saying, "Okay, we will put you in the queue. Likely you'll have surgery in about one and a half years, which is much quicker than it used to be."

Talk about a lifestyle and worldview change!

CHAPTER 31
Patient Grades

During the year the interns saw what they thought were some questionable patient-care decisions. While on surgery rotations with doctors who did elective surgeries, they always wondered if the public should just get doctors' credit scores instead of Healthgrades (grades by other patients) or other online reviews.

Examples of cases for which they scrubbed and scratched their heads included minimal fractures, joint replacements, plastic surgery, endovascular procedures, ingrown fingernails (in the operating room), injections, and dental procedures. Then they would order tests. One of the vascular surgeons would order a battery of tests no matter what the complaint was. If a patient came in with a non-healing ulcer because of blood flow in one leg, he would receive tests for blood flow in both legs, abdominal tests to rule out an aneurysm, and carotids, just to name a few. When asked why he ordered all the tests, the physician said the hospital and he needed the money.

If it was just for billing for tests, that could be allowed. Everyone knew that radiology is the only specialty that can refer to themselves. CT could be many pathologies, and the Radiologist recommends to clinically correlate. They could recommend a patient get an MRI or nuclear medicine studies, which are body scans with contrast die, then their department would get more money. Perhaps these patients needed the additional imaging and it could be justified, but when there was a blurred line and a doctor was known for just buying a sports car or new vacation home, they started to wonder about these trends.

So, the tests occurred, and the vascular surgeon hoped to find something else wrong that he could fix. In other words, he hoped to find asymptomatic pathology so that he could tell the patient they had to fix it. Sometimes they did find urgent or emergent issues, but that wasn't the norm. All of this adds to the financials of the practice and their bonuses. This trend is getting worse. At this large hospital that offers numerous programs, from family practice to neurosurgery training, the average resident physician has just under $400,000 in student loan debt.

Many are unable to make payments, and the amount due continues to grow. This is a lifetime of payments, even on a doctor's salary, and not all will be successful doctors. The loans on average are at 7 percent interest rate. Last year many physicians owed more than $1 million in student loan debt to the government. While physicians try to keep up with the Joneses, they are strapped financially. Perhaps less costly tuition would mean better patient care; however, some folks get into financial trouble even when they win the lottery. Due to insurance cuts, doctors work more, see more patients, do more paperwork, and are paid less than previous doctors. Like Robert, Samantha, and David told each other, they would drive the old pickup trucks in the surgeons' parking lot that was full of sports cars worth hundreds of thousands of dollars. Let the surgical sales reps drive the nice sports cars!

The problem with physicians is the majority are excellent, but a few ruin everyone's reputations. There are a few doctors who, like professional athletes or rock stars, think money doesn't matter and they can outearn their stupidity. The physician thinks they must look a certain way, and in a lot of ways, society supports that mindset. The interns heard patients say all the time during their intern year, "I know he's a great surgeon because he drives a Porsche." The interns would think, "No, he's a broke surgeon who's talked you into this procedure you may or may not need."

Most of the reasons behind overspending on healthcare at a national level are defensive practices. The physician is worried about being sued and losing their medical license. If a patient comes in with a complaint, tests are ordered, which can lead down the rabbit hole to more testing and procedures. Doctors are taught this in school and during residency. Many become cynical, particularly toward government insurers such as Medicaid. Many times, as said before this patient population wants to have all the tests done. If it's free, why wouldn't you want all the tests done? The problem is the taxpayers who fund this don't know about this problem.

This could change if tort malpractice cases were not allowed or if patients could be punished for bringing a bogus claim to the courts. Without those changes, there is no end in sight. Consider this example: During their emergency department rotations, all the interns saw the same patient. He was 42 at the time and neurotic about having cancer. Every day he came into the emergency department with malingering abdominal pains and demanded a CT scan. Yes, virtually every day. On average, for the past few years, he had over 300 CT scans in the chart per year, scans that found nothing except maybe GI air (a fart in motion) or bloating. Robert told the patient, "You don't have cancer now, but if you keep getting radiation every day, it's going to happen!" Meanwhile Robert thought if this patient would just admit to and let us treat his anxiety his life would be more enjoyable, how stressful is waiting in the emergency department every day!

The problem stems from the patient bearing no cost for these tests (because he was on Medicaid) and from the physician's fear that if they don't order the scan and something is wrong, they will be in a lawsuit for the next 5 to 10 years. However, interns were paid a minimal salary, and David needed testing for a suspected bladder infection. He debated (like most of working society does) whether he could afford the cost that his private employer insurance wouldn't cover. David was on the house officer rotation, which is the most difficult month, with a monster of a senior resident who was on a power trip. She was a hardened woman in medicine who had a chip on her shoulder, and he was a young, attractive man who by definition made her mad. So for a month, from the time he arrived at 4:30 a.m. until he left after 6:00 p.m. David wasn't allowed to eat or use the bathroom. This finished when he came down with the bladder infection.

The system bears some blame in overspending on healthcare, but so does the physician, not only for practicing defensive medicine but also for over-testing, trying to drum up business. There is nothing worse than a physician doing unnecessary surgery for financial gain. Most of these physicians get burned and caught when they take a patient in for a minimal procedure and have an anesthesia complication.

Samantha worked with a vascular doctor who took the same patient in for a leg angiogram and intervention, such as stents and balloons, at least once a month for years. In the end, when the attending was caught by the state medical board, the patient's ankle brachial index was still 0.18, which means they had about 18 percent of blood flow in the leg. There was no pain because of neuropathy, but the leg was grey-blue, and had to be amputated.

David always said people should pick their doctors by word of mouth, not by radio or TV ads. Surgery nurses are the most trustworthy as it's a small world. They all talk and know who to trust and who not to trust. Unfortunately, they can't get the word out to the public due to HIPPA concerns and restrictions. After all, a lot of online physician reviews come from competing practices, disgruntled nurses and staff, and the practice themselves to persuade or dissuade consumer patients.

Perhaps we need an open forum where medical staff can be public online regarding providers and patients. Noncompliant patients and doctor shoppers can be identified. Ethical, moral, and outstanding surgeons and practitioners can be mentioned and reviewed. Sadly, we're a long way from this in the United States of America and will have to deal with the current roll-the-dice medical climate!

CHAPTER 32
Pro Prophylaxis

Samantha was an independent, strong woman and a rock star during the intern year—much better than the guys she was with, David and Robert. As a young professional, many of her societal and moral views would be challenged during the intern year, including when she was on emergency department rotation and surgery. The first time Samantha did a speculum exam, which is when a metallic or clear plastic spreading device is inserted into the patient's vagina and spread to visualize their anatomy and take samples for HPV (for example), was on her first day in the emergency department.

She was told to evaluate a patient that frequently came to the emergency department, sometimes stable and sometimes not, after doing a home abortion. The patient was an uneducated female in her 20s, and she had a friend with her. She was moderately obese and had large hoop earrings. She was laughing and having fun with her friend, which could be heard from the hallway. Samantha expected a different type of patient for a failed attempt at an abortion at home, perhaps someone somber and quiet, reserved, maybe ashamed.

Samantha introduced herself and told the patient what to expect. The patient seemed proud to say this was her 17th time coming in for this. She had figured out how to use a clothes hanger when she got pregnant, and when bleeding occurred, she went to the emergency department for removal of the fetus. Samantha could only hear the TV and the patient and her friend laughing. After inserting and opening the speculum, Samantha saw a lifeless fetus. She slid the fetus onto the speculum and out to the mayo stand, a moveable table with a sterile field she had set up.

Samantha went to one of the best colleges in America that had a very liberal campus, and she had always believed a woman had a right to choose what happened to their bodies. She didn't have a political affiliation, but Samantha was a staunch pro-choice defendant and Planned Parenthood volunteer in the past. The small, lifeless fetus was about the size of her palm. It was a male and looked less like an alien and more like a small human being. She looked at the fetus and then at the patient, who didn't have a care in the world. The patient used the emergency department and abortion as contraception.

This shook Samantha, who called Robert, someone she could speak with candidly. Her worldview was rocked. After a lengthy conversation, they both knew this wasn't just a crazy person and that they would see much more of this during their training. However, for babies born to drug-addicted mothers, babies born as a result of rape or molestation, etc., abortion was still okay, wasn't it? Samantha believed there was a place for it.

Then Samantha was on surgery and working with an older attending who made tons of money doing abortions. He estimated he had easily done 5,000 abortions in his career. Samantha was hopeful he would provide insight into the moral compass of this. She was wrong. The attending was doing it for the money, and he felt justified in this practice. After all, it wasn't his choice; it was the patients' choice.

The first true abortion Samantha did was with this attending. It was a simple procedure done in the operating room. Basically, they had to control the bleeding and use an instrument called a Kocher (picture a pair of scissors but the ends are rat-toothed and fit together in grooves. By the handle there are ratchets that interlock. This tool is designed to grab an object and engage the grooves; it won't let go no matter the force applied or the object it grasps.)

Legislation still exists in this country for some states to do late-term abortions. In other words, when, with today's medical technology, a fetus could be born and survive, some physicians are still doing abortions on these fetuses. So there went Samantha, having a whole day ahead of her of late-term abortions: The Kocher goes in, there's a crunch, a twist, and then, with a pull, a small body part is extracted and put on the back table. Starting out, she would grab and feel or hear the crunch and pull back, thinking in her mind, *Well, there's a leg*. The head was the worst. When she grabbed the head, there was usually fight back from the fetus (whether intentional or unintentional, this could be debated), and then the skull would break and cerebral spinal fluid would flow out, the fighting would stop.

At the end of every case, Samantha would look at the sterile field table and put together the limbs, torso, and head (if they were not too mangled) of a tiny human boy or girl. Samantha hadn't slept well since this, and she did have to work with physician's health and wellness as she felt that she murdered numerous humans that day. Worse yet, she murdered humans who couldn't argue or fight back. Lives were lost because of the mothers' rights and their decisions.

It's hard to know when the abortion is too late—is it heartbeat or brain function? Certainly, late-term abortions are against typical

American morals and ethics. Perhaps all abortions are. Who knows who that child could become? There have been drug-addicted infants, infants born in poverty, and children who have suffered abuse who have made great contributions to society.

Samantha wrapped her head around legislation that wasn't about telling women what they could do with their bodies but was about trying to limit questionable murder. Does the world have to be so polarized on political decisions such as this? Can't there be a linear continuum of how we, as society, look at this issue? Samantha spent a lot of time researching and pondering this topic and actually went on to lecture on this subject in the future. Could you be pro-choice when a fetus is eight days old and pro-life when a fetus is eight months old? She thought most people would agree pro-life after birth is a given, but this varies by state. People still feel a fetus can be aborted at birth, particularly if it has defects or for other social or moral reasons.

Samantha gave a tremendous end-of-year research and ethics presentation. As the capstone to the intern year, every intern gives a lecture on a topic of their choosing that is typically related to their research projects and interests. This is done in front of the entire medical staff, other learning physicians, and outside physicians who get continuing medical education credits. Samantha's project fascinated the crowd.

As one attendant commented, "When future generations look back on this time, this will be the most barbaric and savage things human beings have done, and I doubt it will continue in the future."

Samantha agreed that the worst thing health professionals have done is hide these horrific procedures from the patient. They don't look at the mangled fetus; it's simply taken care of. Now

Samantha says she's pro-life and mostly pro prophylaxis—use contraception, not murder, to control the population and to family plan. After all, this was the most influential item for women in our time—family planning with contraceptives and not just having babies, allowing women to be out in the workforce and work towards equality.

CHAPTER 33
Dog-Eat-Dog World

Most emergency departments have an electronic board that simply displays a room number and the patient's chief complaint. On-call residents commonly scout this board for various services, looking for patients known to them or complaints they will get called about. Unfortunately, this causes a lot of anxiety as they may never get called on these patients; that decision is up to the emergency department physician.

Here are some examples to explain the emergency department (ED) board: vaginal trauma will have the OB/GYN residents waiting for a call from the ED in the same way a fractured hip keeps Orthopedic Surgery watching, a toe infection keeps Podiatry watching, hand trauma keeps Plastic Surgery watching, and the list goes on and on.

Now the General Surgery residents covering night call get any odd complaint for evaluation, particularly if there is any trauma. At a Level 1 trauma center, some cases come in the door that you wouldn't believe unless you saw them. Many times, there are crimes involved, and the patients are brought by ambulance. Sometimes they are simply dropped off outside the ED on a busy street turnaround by an unknown person who speeds away in their car to avoid police at the ED. It's not uncommon to walk outside the ED and see people literally being pushed out of the passenger seat and lying on the ground. Fortunately, the staff are used to this, and they run after the patient with a gurney and bring the patient into the ED.

David was on emergency department rotation, covering their nighttime service and searching the board when he came across the strangest complaint he'd seen. The slot read "Bite Dog, Vet Needed." His imagine ran wild. Would he be called and what was he going to walk into? Right at that time, as he was finishing a piece of pizza, his pager was blaring. He looked at the pager, downed a soda, and took off toward the ED. What he was about to see couldn't be explained.

He pulled back the curtain, foam-washed his hands, and his jaw dropped. There in the bed was a man in his early 30s wearing a white tank top … and roughly an 80-pound pit bull. A metal chain collar and leash were stuck around the patient and the dog. This metal—in what was obviously a ferocious encounter—had cold-welded to itself, and they were stuck together.

(It's actually not uncommon for patients to get caught in dog leashes. Robert had a patient who put her dog on a chain outside her house, walked to her car, opened the door, and sat inside. The patient didn't realize the dog's chain had wrapped around her ankle and she shut it in the door. She backed down the driveway, and all of a sudden, she felt a strong pull and pop as her ankle broke in three places with the bone coming out of her skin. She required emergent surgery, and the dog went unharmed.)

David looked closer and saw a significant amount of blood all over the bed and floor with active, oozing bleeding from both the man's groin and the dog's. The staff had been holding pressure on the groin of both the patient and the pit bull. The pit bull had needed a sedative and was blurry-eyed and slow-moving. The patient was in excruciating pain.

David started using irrigation saline and gel foam with thrombin to control the bleeding and get a better look. Although there are veterinarians that have emergent clinics, they're not credentialed to work in hospitals, an issue that caused chaos this night. Somehow the ED physician remembered the plastic surgery senior for the hospital had been a veterinarian prior to going to Vietnam and then to medical school. He wasn't on call, but David called him and pleaded his case. Thankfully, the head of plastic surgery, who was 69 years old and looked ten to twenty years older agreed and headed into the hospital.

The patient had suffered a bite injury to his testicles, but strangely, the pit bull suffered a bite to his testicles as well.

"What happened?" said David.

"Man, I was walking outside my place," the patient replied, "and this pit bull that no one claims to own ran up on me with this collar and leash dragging behind. I decided not to run and tried to make myself big—you know, like scaring a bear. That's when the fucker bit me in the balls. Well, I believe eye for an eye and shit, so I wrapped him up with the leash and bit him in the balls! Man, would you believe no one in the trailer park would help me?"

The patient was wrapped up with the dog, and someone apparently saw this and called the police, who were bedside.

The cop laughed. "It's the strangest thing I've seen," he said. "So, who do we give the rabies shot to—the patient or the dog? Who's infecting who here?"

The plastic surgeon came in, and the cops helped cut the chains to free the patient and the dog. The dog was taken to a 24-hour veterinarian with packing to keep him from bleeding.

The patient went into the operating room with David and the plastic surgeon. He had bleeding and testicular torsion, which is where the anatomic structures wrap around themselves; it can be problematic long term. The patient was then followed by urology. David never saw the patient or the dog again after that night.

CHAPTER 34
When Animals Attack

It was early spring, and the brutal winter landscape was melting away. The trees were coming to life, and it was almost as if people were coming out of hibernation as the days grew longer and warmer in the sunshine. Samantha was on call and had a run of seeing only already admitted patients and answering the never-ending calls of critical lab values and questions from nurses and staff. She thought to herself, *What a beautiful day. Where are all the motorcycle accidents and home repair injuries?* Typically, spring cleaning means a large volume of injured do-it-yourself patients. (This patient type changes to the "hold my beer, watch this" patient type as summer gets into full swing.)

Samantha was heading to the bathroom when she got a page. It was the emergency room doctor who was out of breath and yelling at her to get to the trauma bay. The midlevel provider (meaning a physician assistant or nurse practitioner) got on the phone, and Samantha couldn't follow what she was trying to explain. She heard "tiger" and "house-pet dog" and the name of an affluent woman who was well-known—famous, actually—in the city. Nothing that the physician assistant said made much sense besides the patient was in trauma bay 2, and there was some animal injury. Samantha put off going to the bathroom and briskly walked down to the emergency department trauma bay.

When she arrived, she found the patient (an upper-class woman in her mid-50s) with many injuries, mostly lacerations and puncture-type wounds to all her extremities and her back. Her hair was newly permed, and tears streamed down her face, smearing her makeup. She looked shocked. The patient was bleeding from her mouth and ears, which might indicate head trauma, as well as from her extremities. Interestingly, she was conscious, alert, and oriented x 3, which meant she knew person (who she was), time (what year it was), and place (which hospital).

Samantha had seen a victim of gang violence who looked like this once earlier during her intern year, but why, she wondered, would this particular patient be "jumped" by a group of people? Fortunately, there were no signs of gang rape, which occurred in the patient Samantha had seen before.

The patient kept screaming, "Where is Precious? Is she okay?!" over and over again until Samantha's head was ringing. Because it's not uncommon for patients with this type of trauma, particularly those who remain lucid and haven't lost too much blood, to scream nonsensical comments, the rest of the trauma team thought nothing of it and kept working.

When a patient arrives in the trauma bay, they are immediately stabilized and placed on a table similar to those in the operating room. Large scissors are used to cut off all their clothes, and the naked, injured person lies there and is inspected head to toe— every crevice, orifice, and site—to ensure there is no missed trauma. This systematic approach is used because physicians are all human, and if a bone is sticking out, it's easy to focus on that and miss an important—and even more life-threatening— injury.

All of a sudden, the patient's husband walked into the trauma bay, which is not typical unless the patient has expired, and all is cleaned up; then the family is brought in. Again, her husband was as well-known as she was in the city and hospital, and unfortunately, I think this preference allowed unfair access. The odd thing was the husband was carrying a peekapoo, a dog weighing no more than 10 pounds, whose front legs were wrapped and who had some blood on its fur. Not only is it uncommon for family to come into the trauma bay during an active process, it's even more uncommon for them to be allowed to bring in a pet. As the husband walked up, the patient let out one last "Precious!" and, with a smile on her face, she passed out.

Her vitals remained stable, and she was just hanging on with all the pain until her dog arrived—or so we thought. Indeed, the dog was named Precious. Samantha spoke with the husband in the corner of the trauma bay, and he explained that they had a new neighbor who moved in beside them. He said he was in his late 20s and single, which was a surprise in a gated neighborhood where houses sat on two-acre plots of land. Samantha had gone to a function at a house in that neighborhood for a resident's graduation party, and she knew that the smallest homes were around 10,000 square feet and the rest went up from there. The husband was describing their neighbor as a young professional athlete who had family and friends over intermittently.

Unknown to the patient and her husband, the athlete next door collected wild animals. That morning, his staff and the athlete were washing the animals in the back, and a tiger got loose. As luck would have it, the patient had let Precious out to use the bathroom at the same time. (They had an electric fence that allowed Precious to roam the acreage.) The patient was watching from the back patio when the tiger went flying into the yard. At first, she couldn't believe her eyes and just stood there, shaking her head. The tiger didn't see Precious, so she ran through the house, down the stairs, and to the backyard. By that time, Precious and the tiger were at a standstill. Samantha thought anyone else at that point would have just said goodbye to Precious and run inside and hide.

The husband explained that Precious had belonged to their 17-year-old daughter and that when their daughter passed in a texting-while-driving car accident, Precious came to hold a special place in the patient's heart. The patient ran toward the backyard as the tiger started to pounce, yelling at the cat and trying to distract it. The husband called the police, who summoned the first responders and wildlife team. Fortunately, they arrived in under five minutes to their house. Meanwhile, the patient had gotten between the dog and the tiger and fended off the tiger long enough for the responders to get there. The tiger was shot and killed, and Precious had only minimal injuries.

The husband said the next-door neighbor athlete was being either arrested or fined and that they were seizing all the other exotic animals. Samantha rolled back to the operating room with the attending trauma surgeon and the patient, who was about to undergo a lengthy surgery. It took 14 hours for the first surgery to stabilize the patient, including efforts of the following teams: orthopedic trauma, general surgery trauma, and neurosurgery. The patient lived and returned to a fairly normal life. Of course, she required extensive therapy at home, 24-hour care initially, plastic surgery reconstruction, and additional procedures. She would have a lifetime of pain, but her dear Precious was still alive and well.

An aside about plastic surgery: there are two types, cosmetic and reconstructive, and only a few doctors do well working as both. Typically, this is the new surgeon in a group who is taking hospital calls, and as their practice grows and they become more senior, they go into a specific area. In other words, there are reconstructive plastic surgeons, such as the one who saw this patient, who specialize in trauma and burns. Then there are cosmetic plastic surgeons, who typically do elective surgeries, such as breast reconstructions, tummy tucks, and facial procedures. Remember that there are two different types and choose accordingly, should you ever need their services.

Samantha had worked with a plastic surgeon who fixed a wound after open-heart surgery. They flipped the omentum, a covering over the abdominal wall, on itself, covered the deficit, and then skin-grafted over this. Samantha described having her sphincter tight during the whole case as the patient's heart was beating right under where she was suturing in the graft. That surgeon told her, "Bright lights, cold steel." The surgeon could do almost anything and had an old-school god complex. However, Samantha (and everyone else) knew he could reconstruct but he had no business doing breast implants.

Samantha was in the first six hours of the tiger vs. socialite case before being tagged out by David who was taking over call for her. Exhausted, she went by the physicians' lounge and looked at the TV and then her smartphone. She saw the trending news report about an animal attack and that the patient was in critical condition. By that time, Samantha knew the patient would live; she just didn't know what her function would be afterwards.

Samantha was shocked to see all the animal rights and social justice warriors making comments about how the tiger should not have been shot. She thought, *If you're the one fighting a tiger on your property, wouldn't you want it shot and killed? Or would you want to try and sedate it, making the odds you'll die even higher?*

Everyone's got an opinion until they're staring down a hungry killing machine.

CHAPTER 35
Dog Days of Summer

Near the residents' office and meeting space on the 15th floor of the professional building was a small patio on the roof. It was great place that administration hadn't discovered yet where residents and staff had put a table and chair and made a small sitting area. It offered a great view of downtown and the horizon.

It was a Saturday morning in early fall and still pleasant in the morning. The leaves hadn't started to change color, though the air was crisp and less humid. Robert was just starting his house officer rotation, taking deep breaths on the patio and meditating, thinking about surviving the beginning of the intern year, when his pager began blaring and ringing in his head.

Robert snuck back through the window that opened to allow access back into the building and went to the residents' office phone. He called the emergency department back, and the unit clerk put him on hold. He shook his head, thinking, *I returned the call within 30 seconds, and now I have to wait.*

After a few minutes the emergency department doctor told Robert he'd better hurry down to the emergency department; he had one of the worst shoulder dislocations and fractures he'd seen—high-energy trauma with concern for paralysis and dysvascular changes to the patient's left arm.

Robert went flying down the hallway and frantically pushed the elevator button over and over until the elevator doors opened. As the elevator descended, he impatiently tapped his toe, and when the door opened, he flew to the trauma bay in the emergency department. There he found a pleasant, well-dressed, 78-year-old African American woman whose hair and makeup were done. She was in a lot of pain but very kind to all the staff, and she was alert and oriented. Robert immediately thought she had suffered a fall from height or a high-energy motor vehicle accident.

The humerus was broken with an acute tear of the rotator cuff, which was retracted, and the arm was flopping; she didn't have control of the arm. There was decreased capillary refill time to her fingers with decreased inflow. The humerus was sticking out of the skin, and gauze that had been placed over the bone was wet with blood. There was not much debris at this site, and Robert couldn't understand how both an open fracture in the middle of the bone and a shoulder dislocation could occur. Was the patient abused by someone? Was she hit with a baseball bat?

Robert was able to reduce the fracture and shoulder with the help of the orthopedic trauma fellow. With reduction, the blood flow was restored to the fingers and hand, and her pain decreased as well; however, she still had a neurological deficit. Although this was not as urgent as losing blood flow to the arm, it was still concerning.

Fortunately, the patient was right-hand dominant, so it was her nondominant hand that was injured. Her tetanus was updated, IV antibiotics were started, she was given pain medication, and her arm was stabilized. The plan was to get her to the operating room with the center's excellent orthopedic shoulder surgeon, who was nationally known.

Robert consented the patient for surgery, including open reduction and repair of fracture and joint along with nerve and artery repair and if needed external fixation or even amputation. The left arm and shoulder were a mess and would require multiple surgeries to salvage. Her long-term function may be limited, but the patient had a great outlook and didn't seem fazed. As she went to the pre-operative holding area, she had one important question for Robert.

"Can you have someone help my dog?" the patient said.

Robert replied, "What do you mean?"

The patient then described how her injury occurred, and after hearing the story, Robert thought it could have happened to anyone, plus the interns had already seen a similar injury in another patient with their ankle. The patient got ready to go to the grocery store, and given that it was such a pretty day, she left her German shepherd outside. She had done this before on nice days as no one messed with him and he was on a chain by the driveway. The dog preferred this, and there was less potential for accidents or damage to the inside of her house, which Robert pictured as a nice suburban home for this pleasant patient.

As she had done many times in the past, the patient tied the dog to the chain by the driveway and got into her car. What she didn't realize as she turned the car on, put on her seat belt, and started to back out was that the chain was wrapped around her left arm. She felt a slight pull that she thought was the seat belt as she struggled to turn her body and check behind her so that she could reverse into the street. She was clear, no cars coming either way. She hit the gas and immediately heard loud noises and felt the worst pain she'd ever had in her life.

She had backed the car out of the driveway with the dog chain around her arm. The patient said fortunately her dog was not injured as the chain held and her arm didn't. The stake, the chain, and the dog were relatively unaffected, according to the EMS notes. The chain simply open fractured and dislocated her arm and then broke through the car door. Fortunately, a neighbor saw this happen and called for emergency services. The patient had the wherewithal to pull her car back into the driveway. EMS stopped the bleeding with a tourniquet and stabilized the patient.

The dog had been left on the chain outside throughout this crisis, so before surgery, Robert called the neighbor (whose number he got from the patient), who was more concerned about the patient than the dog. They had an extra key to the house and had already put the dog inside; they would continue to feed and care for the dog. Right before surgery Robert updated the patient, and she was calm going into the operating room.

As Robert worked with the attending shoulder surgeon, they were able to salvage the limb. There would be chronic swelling and the risk for complications, but for now she had the arm. The injury would require staged procedures for soft-tissue repair.

Robert couldn't get out of his mind the love this widowed woman had for her dog. She was more concerned about the dog than losing her arm—or her life, for that matter. Robert had been trained to be objective and cold when it came to emotions; this is important when making decisions about patients' lives. Taught through generations of physicians and surgeons is the theory that doctors can't get caught up in the emotions. However, every physician and surgeon at times fights this mental battle of compassion and sadness for the patient versus the objective science of medicine and surgery.

CHAPTER 36
Freshly Cut

The orthopedic department had a national reputation for being a center of excellence, and they prided themselves on their outcomes and providing efficient care without mistakes. As humans and doctors, we are truly scientists and know that mistakes happen and that it's best to learn from them so that we can improve. Even as interns, we constantly checked and balanced ourselves in a never-ending game of "What could have been better?" and "What could have been worse?" "What could we have done differently?" and "How do we learn from this?" A doctor lives a life of checks and balances coupled with lifelong learning.

Samantha was assigned to a committee required to have a resident's presence, and they reviewed what we refer to as "sentinel events" at the hospital, events for which there is no discussion of appropriateness and it's black-and-white wrong or inappropriate care. Even if it's an honest mistake, it is reported to the national boards and issue-reviewed, and a record is kept of it. Sometimes it's a near miss and no patient is harmed, while others are disastrous, and the patient is harmed or dies. Then there are those we couldn't make up if we tried that are hilarious. As you can imagine, these are few and far between. In a Level 1 trauma center, you would be surprised to see one every five to ten years.

Samantha called David and Robert immediately after the meeting. She had signed a silly nondisclosure agreement for the committee to not speak about events. However, she didn't need to use doctor or patient information to tell this story, and she knew it would quickly spread across the hospital like wildfire.

She called David from her cell phone then patched in Robert as a conference call. "Guys, you won't believe what happened in the pre-op area today!"

Pre-operative bays 30 and 31 each held a 74-year-old Caucasian patient with nondescript names, and the anesthesia techs (in the past referred to as orderlies) were assigned to prepare the patients This included transport to the operating room, setting up for surgeries, shaving the patients, preparing equipment, running to get odds and ends requested, and helping direct families.

Typically, patients are grouped by service line and time of arrival, meaning neurosurgery patients in one area and vascular surgery patients in another and so on. However, earlier in the day bay 30 held a urology patient and bay 31 held a total knee-replacement patient. David and Robert could start to see what happened as she described the event.

The anesthesia tech, a 19-year-old, high-energy, one-year-out-of-high-school, cocky former jock mixed the patients up. The damn thing was the patients didn't know any better and didn't say anything. The mix-up was missed until they got into the operating room. The correct patients ended up in the correct operating rooms, but there was a different oversight that the interns couldn't believe.

The anesthesia tech shaved the testicles of the total knee-replacement patient and the knee of the urology patient. The 74-year-old gentlemen patients just assumed it was protocol.

David said, "I get the urology patient saying nothing about the knee shaving, but what the hell was the knee-replacement patient thinking about his balls being shaved?!"

Samantha said the patient stated that he assumed it was a new-age protocol, and he didn't mind his hedges being trimmed and knee being replaced!

Surgery sites are shaved to avoid cysts, infection, reactions, and complications with surgery. Although this was a reportable sentinel event, no one was harmed, and the patients didn't file a complaint.

Samantha said, "Yep, some old guy got a story to tell his friends—a free shave and a new knee!"

CHAPTER 37
Mom Knows Best

The interns had a renowned residency program director, which is the attending senior physician in charge of the residency program who is typically academically focused and organized, as well as willing to miss some clinical work with patient care for administration. With a large residency program, there are over 50 attending surgeons of all specialties. David was assigned to cover elective surgeries, which this month included surgeries done by all of the specialist and taking care of their patients during the post-operative hospital stays.

Surgeries covered by the interns include pain cases, such as injections and spinal stimulators; podiatry (foot and ankle surgeries); plastic surgery; orthopedics, including joint replacements; vascular surgery; endocrine surgery; ear, nose, and throat cases; general surgery; and the list goes on and on. This assignment requires a constant study of texts, journal articles, and online resources to stay current with each specialty, not only from the standpoint of surgery technique but also post-operative treatment, particularly when in the hospital.

David was scheduled to do a long day of foot and ankle surgeries with a well-respected, upbeat, funny podiatrist. Many of the interns wished they'd gone into this field because of the hours and pay; however, the work was harder than they thought. This young attending was liked by the residents and fellows, and particularly by the female nurses and staff.

However, he was a devoted family man with young children. There were 16 surgeries that day, and only three would need to be admitted. Midway through the day, the podiatric surgeon told David he really didn't want to do this bunion and ankle repair surgery.

With elective cases, attendings talk about "their Spidey sense": if they spot a "problem patient" before surgery, they avoid the procedure if possible (of course this doesn't apply to traumas or infection surgeries; no attending would turn down a patient who needed urgent or emergent care). In the case of elective surgeries, which was the kind of case David was about to start, many times conservative care, second opinions, and alternatives to surgery are employed to avoid a "problem patient." Each attending surgeon describes a problem patient differently, such as needy, overly questioning, not reliable to follow post-op care, and noncompliant.

David asked the attending why he didn't want to do this relatively straightforward outpatient, elective surgery. The attending explained he was the fourth opinion to see this patient. She reported exhausting conservative treatments, but he knew this wasn't true. However, you can only go off what the patient tells you, particularly when they don't sign the consent to release medical records from other physicians' offices. He tried to convince her to try conservative care that might have decreased her symptoms. He discussed risk and outcomes long-term with the patient, who always had her children—a teenager and pre-teen—at the office appointments. Once the attending agreed to surgery, he usually booked the procedure about a month out, but this patient bullied her way with the surgery scheduler and added on that week, in addition to pushing the hospital to perform pre-surgery testing and get scheduled.

Although reluctant to do it, the surgeon performed this procedure masterfully. It was straightforward without an issue and took just under 45 minutes. A splint was applied, and when the patient woke up from anesthesia without incident, she was taken to the post-anesthesia care unit (PACU). When she woke up, she complained of excruciating pain, even though she had a nerve block before surgery (meaning the anesthesia doctor gave her an injection of local anesthetics above her knee that typically numbs the leg for around 12–24 hours). David asked the anesthesiologist if there was obvious pain during surgery, and they reported all vitals and signs suggested the patient could not feel her extremity and hadn't required much additional anesthesia to remain unconscious.

The patient continued to be in pain, and her children were the family in the recovery area. Typically, this area is for adults only, for the caregivers, but there was no other family—just the patient's gangly 16-year-old and 12-year-old sons. David was told to admit the patient for 23 hours for observation— essentially an overnight in the hospital covered by insurance for outpatient observation. The patient and her children were taken upstairs for admission and care by the floor team and staff. This was all uneventful, and no red flags were raised.

Samantha came on overnight, and at least once an hour she received a page or direct call on this patient for post-operative pain. It didn't make sense; a bunion and ligament repair at the ankle didn't usually require this much oral and intravenous opioids to control pain. Samantha called David in the morning and told him that since she'd been up all night dealing with this patient, he'd better have an answer for what he did to the patient in surgery; she wanted him to round on the patient with her this morning. When they walked into the room, the 16-year-old was sleeping on the couch that folds into a bed against the window and back wall of the patient room. The 12-year-old was sleeping in the bed beside his mother. There were numerous bags of clothes and food scattered throughout the room.

The patient had the splint on, and she had no problems with therapy using the crutches and staying off her foot. However, when asked about her pain level, she would reply she was feeling 10/10.

David said, "Honey, people who are 10/10 pain are writhing in pain and on fire. If the medication we're giving you isn't working, we need to stop the opioids and try something else." This was the line David had learned to use to deal with patients who were opioid-dependent and just drug-seekers. They would beg to keep the opioids going and change their story.

However, this patient was different. She said, "You can change to whatever medication you want. I'm just in too much pain to go home today and need to stay longer."

The next day Samantha and David rounded, and it was the same routine, except this time the 16-year-old had left with the 12-year-old for school and wouldn't return until the afternoon. The patient didn't feel safe going home and wanted to stay in the hospital. This went on for another week. The nurses noticed that the patient was eating minimally and asking for additional food from the fridge, dividing most of the food with her boys. At first, the nurses thought they were being helpful; then they realized that she was just feeding her children through the nurses' kindness.

After the week's stay in the hospital, the social worker was asked to discuss with the patient the fact that the insurance carrier would not cover the majority of her stay, nor any future stay. This could lead to hundreds of thousands of dollars billed directly to the patient and would mean certain bankruptcy for almost anyone.

The patient wasn't fazed by this one bit. She stayed true to her comments that her pain wasn't being addressed, and she refused to go home in such pain. The attending surgeon had been seeing her daily and asked David and Samantha on morning rounds to step out. He wanted to speak with the patient alone. After about 10 minutes the attending surgeon walked out of the patient's room and into the hallway.

The surgeon's instincts were correct. The woman reported being homeless shortly before surgery, and she and her children were living in her car. She had too much pride to ask for help and thought that if she could be admitted to the hospital, they would have a place to stay and food to eat, buying her time to figure out her next steps. She also hoped that her family would feel sorry for her if she were hospitalized and help her and the children.

The patient explained she was a former heroin addict and that her husband was incarcerated for heroin possession. He had been an accountant at a large firm, and she was an intern in college. They met, and she eventually joined the firm. For years they lived a good life in the suburbs: The kids went to private schools. They had a mortgage, credit cards, and cars. They were essentially "normal."

The brother of the patient's husband was released from prison, and they were the only ones who would take him in. That was where they went wrong. The brother got her husband hooked on pain pills and eventually heroin. She tried it once and was hooked. Years later, here they were. The kids were in public school and barely showing up, and she was a recovering addict, living in a hospital room on the fourth floor without any resources or hope for a better future.

Immediately the social worker started helping the mother and her children. Behavioral health was consulted, and the patient was transferred from the medical/surgical floor to the psychiatric ward. She had a mental break and put herself at risk when her children needed her the most. The children's grandparents did indeed show up, took the children to their house, and took over their care and education.

The last Samantha heard, they were working on becoming legal caretakers for the children, and the attending told David the patient was healing. The surgery had gone great as expected; she was back to walking pain-free and fitting into shoes. She was also in a single-mother rehabilitation facility, getting help so that she could return to her life and hopefully be with her children eventually. In healthcare we describe heroin addicts as being in remission when they are not using, just like a cancer patient, meaning they are clean now but could use again at any time.

David told Samantha, "For everyone's sake, let's hope the husband stays in jail and can't make any of this worse." Samantha simply shook her head.

CHAPTER 38
Keep on Grinding

Robert was two weeks into the orthopedic trauma rotation, lower than a rookie surgeon and trying to do his best for patients as he was surrounded by hardworking, brilliant orthopedic surgeons and a traumatologist.

Robert's biggest learning point was the "tattoo-to-teeth ratio," a common saying in the trauma world that Robert had already seen to be accurate after only a short time on this service. The saying meant that if the patient had more tattoos than teeth, they would survive almost anything. There may be prejudice in this, but it was fact, and working at a Level 1, downtown hospital he was seeing this firsthand. There seemed to be evolutionary differences among socioeconomic classes based not on race, gender, or religion but on this fact: the harder life you've had, the more you can survive.

In only a couple weeks he'd seen patients with more tattoos than teeth survive 50-foot falls from trees, 70+-mile-per-hour car crashes that flipped, and being shot multiple times; the patients not only survived these incidents, they quickly recovered. Robert had also seen well-kept, middle-age attorneys, accountants, and teachers slip and fall at home, or off a curb, or at a restaurant and die in the trauma bay—or even en route to the hospital. Robert also learned that patients with misspelled tattoos or rose tattoos with names in them were almost indestructible. When one of these patients survived a horrendous injury and were asked where they got the tattoos, it wasn't uncommon to hear that they did the tattoos themselves or got them in prison.

While working this rotation, Robert had a 45-year-old female patient who worked at a mulch company. One day a week her job was to clean the mulch grinder, a large device that she climbed into with the help of a ladder and lift. Apparently, it was standard protocol to turn this machine off with a push-button remote control instead of turning it off at the power supply or with a breaker. It turns out she had cleaned this machine several hundred times without issue in the years she had worked there (which makes one wonder if perhaps the more we do something, the less we pay attention as it becomes commonplace).

The blades and devices that turned over the mulch so that it didn't catch on fire were stopped, and there was a minimal amount of mulch at the bottom. When she stepped off the ladder into the bottom of the grinder, she bumped her leg where the remote control was in her pocket and activated the machine. Imagining this situation, you would think she was immediately killed. Although the machine broke her ribs and legs in multiple places, her bones actually stopped the blades and stuck, jamming the machine. She was bleeding but alive.

Immediately the owner of the mulch company called 911. As luck would have it, the helicopter pilot was working his last day prior to retirement with his regular team that consisted of himself and two nurses. However, a friend of his who had been with him in Vietnam wanted to do a ride-along on the last day. (The helicopter pilot had been a bush pilot flying helicopters in Vietnam, and his war friend was a retired Flight Surgeon who, after 25 years in the military, became a trauma surgeon in the civilian world.)

The helicopter landed, and the machine was turned off. The staff hadn't reversed the blades as they didn't want to dislodge them and make it worse or have them spin again on the patient. It turns out this was the best thing they could have done as the pressure of the large blades had helped to stop some of the bleeding. The team from the helicopter climbed in and started to work. The trauma surgeon cauterized (burned) or clamped with a hemostat all the arterial bleeds. They used thrombin and gel foam to stop the bleeding with pressure and stabilized the host of fractures. She had a punctured lung, and the trauma surgeon dropped an airway and chest tube into the patient, which isn't typically done in the field.

She was stabilized and lifted by helicopter to our emergency department. Robert met the patient en route to the trauma bay to get an accurate history of what happened to the patient and, and they were rushed into the operating room. Robert felt his blood pressure go through the roof. His forehead was sweating, his hands were mildly shaking, and his mind was running wild as his heart stuck in his throat. He knew the patient was in poor condition, and any mistake in the operating room would lead to her death. Although no one would be blamed if the patient couldn't be saved as the odds were against her, Robert wanted to do his best. Even when physicians can't win the battle or fix what's wrong with the patient, we continue to push and try to heal until we have exhausted every option—as well as ourselves. For this reason, physicians (who are human too) have many sleepless nights.

"You need to snap out of it or get out of here!" the attending trauma surgeon said to Robert.

Robert looked at the surgeon and could tell by his eyes that he was smiling under the mask.

The attending then said, "Look at the patient's right leg. See how that's spelled? This lady will survive anything."

Robert looked at the mangled extremity. (Remember, she had open fractures to all her extremities and chest wounds.) She had tattoos all over, including sleeves on both arms. She had poor dentation and few normal-looking teeth. As Robert looked down at the leg, he saw a tattoo inked in bold and underlined that said BELEIVE IN YOURCELF.

The attending was right—two misspelled words in one tattoo. This patient would survive anything. And she did. She may have lifelong pain and deformity, but she's alive and rehabbing, walking on her own.

CHAPTER 39
Anger Management

As a Level 1 trauma center, the hospital is required to have certain surgeons on staff and available at all times. Thus, there are several different operating room areas. The main operating room has over 50 surgery suites. Then there is the orthopedic surgery site in another building on campus, a neurosurgery site in yet another building, a heart and endovascular procedure site, and finally, gastroenterology suites as well.

Robert was paged to the orthopedic center for a patient down in the lobby. Typically, this is an overhead page for a code blue, in other words for a patient down and near death or already dead, and members of this team start running when they hear the code.

Robert received instead a simple page from the front desk in the orthopedic lobby, so he walked from one building to another through the basement. (There is a lower level 1 with offices, cadaver lab training, and a pharmacy, and then there is a lower level 2, which is the sub-basement used only for staff traffic. It can be crowded but much quicker than walking through the regular hospital. Additionally, it's a way for doctors and staff to avoid running into patients or other community people they know, which slows down their efficiency. Overall, it's used in the winter to avoid problems between buildings and for disaster preparation.)

Robert arrived in the lobby only to have apparently missed all the action. A hospital security guard was lying on the ground, awake and with an apparent broken nose. Other security guards had a gigantic middle-aged man with a large beard, wearing overalls and a farmer's cap, up against the wall as they placed handcuffs on him. As he watched, Robert couldn't get past the intense malodor permeating the lobby. This was the surgery waiting lobby, and people who were waiting for loved ones who were in surgery were standing in one corner of the lobby, huddled up, with most of them holding their shirts over their face and nose to avoid the stench.

Robert looked to the opposite corner near the front desk and saw the cleaning crew cleaning feces and urine off the floor. *No wonder there's such a disgusting smell*, Robert thought, and then put it out of his mind. With the aid of the police, he helped get the bleeding security guard to a stretcher in preparation for transporting him to the next building's emergency department. The security guard was fine; he held a rag on his face with his head lifted, trying to apply pressure and decrease bleeding.

As the security guard was wheeled down the hall, Robert called over to the emergency department to give them a heads-up and to request topical thrombin and packing with imaging. Certainly, the security guard would be getting some PTO (paid time off), making sure he didn't have a concussion.

The cleaning crew was now focused on cleaning up blood and sterilizing the area. The front desk check-in staff for surgery now included the security guard from the floor below, where there was an overflow surgery waiting area, and the regular desk attendant. Robert ran into Larry, a custodian he'd known since he was a student at the hospital prior to residency, and Larry nonchalantly explained what happened.

"It's not the first time and won't be the last time I see something like this," said Larry. "You've got to understand us humans—we're just socialized animals!"

This is the story Larry told Robert: The man wearing the overalls and hat who was arrested was the husband of a surgery patient who was having a hip replacement performed by one of the hospital's leading orthopedic surgeons. Prior to the surgery, the husband was told to expect the procedure to take about one to one and a half hours. When two hours went by, the patient's husband got anxious, which is a common reaction. Many times, a nurse calls the family from the operating room via the front desk to give an update explaining the delay.

(Imagine you are waiting for a family member to undergo a procedure under anesthesia, and as the hours go by, you hear overhead pages saying, "stroke alert" or "code blue." You start to become anxious. In the operating room, time flies, and the staff isn't always aware there's been a delay because numerous reasons can back up a surgery start time.)

Instead of letting his mind run wild, the patient's husband angrily approached the front desk, asking what the problem was. He said he had a schedule to keep and asked why the doctor and hospital didn't respect his time. The front desk staff did their best to diffuse the man's anger; he sat down but continued to steam. Security was secretly alerted and asked to make rounds in case the situation became worse.

Another 15 minutes went by, and the patient's husband came back up to the desk saying he couldn't wait much longer and needed an update. The front desk called the operating room and were told everything was fine; there were no issues, and they should be done soon. That message was reported to the patient's husband, who sat down and became belligerent, cursing and yelling. Security then arrived and asked the man to calm down.

"You can't tell me what to do," said the husband. "My wife has been in surgery more than an hour beyond the scheduled time."

The security guard started to explain to the patient's husband about delays and that he couldn't cause a scene. That was when the husband stood up and punched the security guard in the face. The security guard went down.

The patient's husband walked over in front of the intake desk and said, "Here's your survey and online review." Then he pulled down his overalls and defecated on the lobby floor.

According to Larry, it was like a train wreck. The other people in the lobby couldn't keep themselves from staring as they let out a collective "Eww." As the patient's husband pulled his overalls back on, the police showed up and arrested him.

Robert said, "Larry! You've seen this before?!"

Larry replied, "I've seen worse, kid, and you will too. I'll tell you some more stories if you ever make it to spin class at the gym."

Robert thought to himself, *I've got to make it to the gym for spin class.*

The gym was a beautiful 5,000-square-foot facility on the top floor of the hospital that offered great city views and all the equipment and a running track anyone could need. Robert used to go, but he couldn't stand the locker rooms. A set of dinosaurs hung out there. By "dinosaurs" Robert meant physicians who should have retired a long time ago, mostly cardiologists who would sit on a leather couch in the locker room completely naked, reading newspapers and academic journals and talking to each other like nothing abnormal was happening. Robert couldn't stand seeing a group of 70-something-year-old men naked on a leather couch, so he ran away.

Robert heard that some of the doctors had indeed finally retired—or perhaps were tapped on the shoulder, told they were practicing antiquated medicine, and asked to resign. Either way, Robert thought he'd give the gym and spin class with Larry a shot. He might just learn something!

CHAPTER 40
Squatters' Rights

It was an odd Midwest spring day early in May with the sun shining and snow falling. Samantha had been an intern for more than 10 months and was on the house officer service when a 58-year-old male drug addict with multiple medical conditions came into the hospital. As it happened, each of the interns spent time caring for this man during the year; his name was commonly on the board and discussed at rounds. The patient was cared for by a primary care physician who still provided hospital care for his patients. (At this Level 1 trauma center, there is a primary care team consisting mostly of internal medicine and family practice physicians who have done hospitalist training.)

This primary care physician was considered "old school," he too was a dinosaur, meaning he did not practice the normal standard of care and protocol. He was the only primary care physician the interns knew of in the city who provided hospital care for their patients.

Well, you can't be two places at once, so if you're seeing patients in your office, the inpatients for whom you're responsible are being cared for by nurses and residents. This physician would try to round in the evenings and write minimal notes, adding comments to the resident's notes from the day. Without the residents, he would not have been able to do this.

The residents enjoyed this. They took pride in caring for these patients as they knew they were directing all their care, not the attending physician. Samantha felt like she had made improvements in this unfortunate man's health and decided she would discharge the patient. After discussing it with the patient, who was in agreement, she put in the discharge orders. A couple hours went by, and she assumed that he left the hospital after nurses reviewed his paperwork and showed him out.

However, two hours after putting in the orders, Samantha was called by the emergency department to see the patient. He had agreed to being discharged and wanted to walk himself out. He took the elevator to the first floor and went immediately to the nursing triage desk. The emergency department brought him in and consulted the attending physician, for whom Samantha was covering. She reviewed the chart on the computer system prior to seeing the patient, trying to wrap her head around why he would be up for readmission after just being discharged. Couldn't the emergency department staff see this in the computer system? She decided to delve deeper into his chart.

After reviewing the patient's record, she was blown away by what she found. Always a self-described nerd at heart, Samantha started writing down chart-note days, including admit and discharge dates. The electronic medical records were a new system as of four years ago, so that was as far back as she could go. As she scrolled through numerous notes, she realized this patient had never left the hospital. He had lived at the hospital for at least four years, and if the records had gone back farther to paper charts, it was hard to tell how long he had been there.

One report did reveal he was discharged about a year prior and left for about three hours. Apparently, he was picked up by his friends, went on an alcohol and cocaine binge, and came in as an overdose. He was immediately admitted to ICU. Other than that occurrence, it didn't appear he'd left the hospital for anything other than to take a smoke break. Samantha initially thought (naïvely) that the patient must think this was terrible, that he must have felt like a prisoner of the health system.

When she pulled back the curtain in the emergency room bay, the patient was not there. He was nowhere to be found in the emergency department. A nurse who had literally just celebrated 50 years of working in the emergency department at this hospital and had actually gone to nursing school at the hospital when she was 18 years old looked at Samantha and said, laughing, "Looking for Bernie?!" Samantha said she was, appearing puzzled, and the nurse said, "Why don't you try the fifth-floor nurses' station."

Samantha went to the elevator and headed to the fifth floor, wondering why in the world the patient being worked up for admit in the emergency department would be on the fifth floor. The elevator dinged, the door opened, and she stared straight at the nursing station. There near the coffee machine stood her patient in a hospital gown.

Samantha walked up to Bernie and said, "Why are you up here on five?"

The patient smirked and said, "Because they have the best coffee on this floor!"

Samantha just shook her head.

The patient was willing to walk back to the elevator and emergency department. However, he told Samantha it was a real treat to be admitted to the fifth floor because of the young, beautiful nurses and the great coffee. He requested admit to that floor.

While riding down and walking back to the emergency room bay, the patient educated Samantha on the healthcare system. You see, Bernie was rather intelligent and savvy. He had gone through a horrible divorce about ten years prior, the kind steeped in hatred. He lost his kids to his ex-wife, an all-too-common scenario when you can't afford an attorney. He had been working as a machinist and representing himself. After this occurred, Bernie left the $18-an-hour job and came to the hospital, first for depression with an admit to the behavioral health unit, and then he saw an opportunity.

He went home and eventually returned to the hospital under the previously mentioned primary care physician's service, the physician who wasn't available at all times to see hospital patients. So, Bernie called the transfer center and ordered a direct admit for abdominal pain under the physician's name and himself as the patient. He checked in at the desk and went into the room. For five days—yes, days not hours—Bernie called verbal orders into the unit clerk on the floor acting as staff from the primary care doctor's office. The verbal orders were placed and left in his chart for the attending to sign. Bernie ordered labs, medications (such as antibiotics), his home medications, and pain medications. He had both a CT and MRI. He even consulted the gastroenterologist to see him through a verbal order. Everyone was charting in the paper chart except for the primary attending, which wasn't caught.

On the fifth day, Bernie ordered morphine and mistakenly ordered a lot of it—"one gallon of mo'phine stat!"—to be exact. The nurse taking the verbal order and the pharmacy both caught this. Security intervened, and of course, the primary attending didn't know he was there and hadn't rounded on him. The police were involved as was administration from the tower. The suits the interns typically despise showed up because this

214

would have been bad PR if it got out. No charges were filed, and the patient wasn't discharged. He was simply transferred to the behavioral health unit for a longer stay.

That's where Bernie said he decided he liked this hospital. It offered a sanctuary from the scary, unsure, dog-eat-dog outside world. So, for the better part of the past decade, he never left.

"After all," he told Samantha, "the food's free, there's maid service, and you can even have your butt wiped by someone else if you ask them to do it. Young, beautiful women speak to you and are kind, which would never happen in the real world. The heat and the AC always work. You get pain medication, and if you're worried you might be dying, you get immediate help," he said, going on and on.

Samantha tried to pick her jaw up off the floor as she walked to the nurses' station at the emergency department to write up his chart and once again admit this patient to the hospital, and of course she requested the fifth floor!

CHAPTER 41
If You're Not First, You're Okay

David was charged with carrying the code pager and being part of the code team, which meant responding to codes and what are referred to as "septic alerts." Various codes can be called overhead throughout the hospital, such as for a fire, a terrorist threat, an abduction, etc., but the "code team" refers to code blues, meaning an actively dying patient. The septic alerts are patients with sepsis, meaning they are showing systemic signs of infection or illness that are life-threatening. David found the septic alerts to be no more than a nuisance, and he hoped he would not be called for a code blue.

David was studying a journal on trauma surgery in the library when "Code blue and hospital room" was announced on the overhead speaker repeatedly. He threw down the journal, gathered his belongings, and took off running as his code pager started blaring. David felt his heart racing—not from running but from anxiety. He expected by the time he got there the work would already be started (typically, respiratory techs, nurses, anesthesia, and others are on the team), or else he'd discover it was a false alarm. As luck would have it, David was the first person to arrive besides a frantic new nurse who was yelling at the patient and doing a sternal rub to wake them.

Immediately after seeing a flatline on the monitor, David started doing chest compressions, which he'd been taught on a mannequin; he had also run scenario codes before. What he didn't realize learning on mannequins (and singing the Bee Gees song "Stayin' Alive" to keep the rhythm of the chest compressions) was the force required. He could feel the ribs break beneath his hands and detach from the patient's sternum in order to be deep enough to be effective. When the team arrived, David started barking out orders for someone to record and others to administer drugs and for respiratory to work on the airway.

Fortunately, the respiratory tech was seasoned and had been working in the hospital for over 35 years; he helped calm David. The respiratory tech had won numerous awards for service and even for patient compassion. The interns and residents used to joke that it was easy for him to win awards—he was helping people to either come back to life or simply breathe better while in the hospital. If you gave someone a breathing treatment when they were gasping, you too would be given an award. However, David quickly realized the respiratory tech was well-known not for silly reasons like these but because he was just as skilled as a physician in a code and had done thousands of them in his career.

Thankfully the anesthesia provider and internal medicine doctor walked in and started to run the code blue. David was now short of breath from the physical exhaustion of running the code and doing chest compression, so a team member tapped him out and continued compressions. The patient survived, was transferred to ICU, intubated, and eventually recovered, making it to the regular floor prior to discharge.

David would become known as a "white cloud" to his intern class as he did the most codes and had the most success during the year. Unbelievably, he was even involved in a code during surgery, during which he immediately started chest compressions. Perhaps it was the depth and the breaking of the ribs, but this patient survived as well. One morning, he was rounding on a very benign mid-70s patient whose daughter was sitting in a chair bedside the bed when the patient went into asystole—his heart stopped beating. David hit the nurses' button and yelled at them for a code blue. He started chest compressions and had the student with him bag (use a squeezable device to insert oxygen into the airway) the patient. The patient lived, and his daughter lived through the trauma of seeing that occur.

Samantha, on the other hand, was more of "black cloud"; she didn't have such luck in codes or on call. She continued to have more and more consults and patient issues; however, she was the intern most equipped to handle these.

Samantha's first code was a disaster. She was carrying the code pager and heard the overhead announcement. She had excelled in running the mock codes in school and during pre-residency training for the hospital system. The knowledge was there, and she was a physician beyond her years, maturity-wise.

She arrived, and all personnel were there—except it was the middle of the night and it was obvious that everyone except the nurses had been asleep in call rooms. The family was present, so they were escorted out to the hallway. Samantha walked into a lot of commotion. The patient was turning blue from lack of perfusion but was alert and awake. The respiratory tech was trying to get oxygen into this obese patient who had multiple medical problems—including COPD, chronic obstructive pulmonary disease—so breathing was already an issue.

Then the patient went into asystole and was no longer awake and alert. Samantha checked for a pulse, and it was absent. She started the code, assigning members of the team to various roles. The anesthesiologist was called, but they were in an emergent C-section at the same time; Samantha would be the only physician. This was no problem. She initially called for epi (epinephrine) which is designed to get a rush to the heart and make it start to contract again. Paddles had been prepared as well. Then the unthinkable happened.

The pharmacist said out loud, "You have got to be shitting me!"

Samantha inquired urgently, and the pharmacist explained that whoever signed off on the crash cart (a wheelable cart that has a digital lock and is full of everything needed for a code blue, including medications) made a deadly mistake. There were no drugs. During a code there isn't time to put in an order and wait for pharmacy to deliver or tube to the nurses' station and then administer it. Seconds count, and the crash cart should have all the drugs needed to run a code—with excess in case it goes longer. Every crash cart has a full stock and is signed off except this one wasn't. There was no epinephrine or other medications readily available.

Samantha did her best. She intubated the patient, and respiratory worked on oxygen while she instructed to continue chest compressions. Another crash cart was obtained, and imaging was being done bedside. Plans for the operating room were made, and the attending surgeon and anesthesia were now in the room. However, those precious seconds were gone. With an anoxic brain, regardless of whether they had been able to keep the patient alive, the patient would have been a vegetable the rest of their life. In this case, they were not able to keep the patient alive. Again, we're all human, but a simple overlook can trickle down to life and death for a patient.

Robert was a mixture of a white and black cloud as some shifts were good and others terrible. However, he did have a knack for getting newly diagnosed cancer patients, and on medicine-attending rotations, he would have to break the news of cancer to a family. Robert was meticulous about making sure the diagnosis was correct; you don't want to just start throwing around the "C" word unless you know for sure. Some doctors inappropriately throw that word around to patients and family ("Well, it looked like cancer") before they know for sure. There is a way to have bedside manner and tact; you certainly don't want to keep the potential of cancer from patients, but you also don't want to give them a diagnosis until it's confirmed by imaging or pathology. Attendings will tell patients they have cancer, and then, when they say, "It's not cancer," patients are pleased. However, the interns didn't believe in this; they thought they should tell patients they have a possibility of cancer but that it could be something else, then break the news if the diagnosis is confirmed.

The joke at our hospital was Robert told more patients they had cancer than the Oncologist did. (Of course, we typically bring in oncology after the diagnosis.) Robert would set the stage by bringing in a chair and making sure the family members were there with the patient. He would try to look each person in the eye while talking, making contact with each of them. He did his best with statistics, which he was always asked about (please remember, though, that 80 percent of statistics are made up on the spot—including the 80 percent just quoted!). He always referred the patient to the counselors, clergy, and other resources. The hardest part today is explaining the hurry-up-and-wait nature of treatment. Patients and their families think that now that the cancer has been found, we're going to start treating it immediately.

Many times, treatments are initiated right away; however, they are long-standing and can take place over years. There is no immediate answer or same-day fix; it requires a team of physicians and a coordinated effort with the patient and their family. Depending on the cancer, sometimes treatment may not even be recommended; the next step may be either watchful waiting or palliative care. Patients want a definitive plan, which the medical professionals certainly understand. The watchful waiting is the worst to handle mentally.

The reality is that every word Robert said after "cancer" was typically forgotten by the patient, which is why he requested family members be present. The patient usually checks out mentally and starts to think about their mortality. The secret is to engage the family if you can, though they are usually taken aback and worried and stop listening as well.

Not everything in life can be predicted. As the physician and the patient, we all must do our best with the hand we're dealt. Studies show none of us make it out of this life alive! Make the most of every day, and try to quickly find inner peace.

CHAPTER 42
Pain in the Ass

There was a Podiatry intern on rotation with Robert and assigned to the house officer shift and surgical service. The Podiatry residents at Robert's facility are truly surgeons. Although Robert wasn't sure if there were different types of Podiatry residencies, these doctors spent the same hours Robert and the other interns spent in the hospital and took on the same responsibilities of patient care. This means that your loved one could be in the ICU with a Podiatry resident managing, say, their vent settings.

The intern asked Robert if he would take a look at a patient who had been in the emergency department for three straight days with hemorrhoid pain—a somewhat common complaint in the emergency department (per the Attendings). Once patients know the diagnosis, however, they usually treat it on their own and don't return. On this patient's third visit, they decided to admit him for a workup—and frankly, a behavioral health evaluation, thinking he just wanted rectal exams. (Honestly, patients have had stranger requests.)

During mid-morning rounds, the attending surgeon, the intern, and Robert walked into the patient's room, the patient being a 26-year-old, seemingly normal male in good shape physically. He reported being an avid weight lifter, which immediately made the doctors think it was a hemorrhoid from straining. They examined his rectum, saw what looked like an inflamed hemorrhoid, and discussed topicals and outpatient follow-up. The patient refused this plan, saying he was concerned about infection because it just showed up and was really painful.

The attending surgeon said to the interns, "Look, the guy's a wimp. That's why he's addicted to weight lifting. Just ask colorectal to take a look before sending him home since the patient says he'll just go to the competing hospital if doesn't get treatment or surgery." (When patients want surgery, that's usually a red flag of a psychiatric issue.)

A CT scan was ordered, which showed only thickening of the tissue and no drainable fluid collection. Robert and the Podiatry intern then saw the patient with the colorectal surgeon who was 51 years old and known for his work ethic, lack of personality, and his resemblance to a vampire—likely due to the fact that he always worked. He was short with his patients and had no bedside manner; however, he was incredibly skilled as a surgeon. He had no tolerance for this patient and quickly said, "We're going to leave and be right back to fix the problem."

Walking into the hallway, he turned to Robert and the other intern and said, "Give the man what he wants. Stick a blade in it." We knew this would be a painful procedure to do bedside; plus, hemorrhoids tend to bleed and can be dramatic, so we prepared for a bleeding hemorrhoid with thrombin and topicals.

Robert walked back into the room and told the patient the plan. The patient lay in a prone, facedown position and lifted the gown. Robert saw an angry hemorrhoid perianal. There was inflammation around the hemorrhoid as well. Injection of local anesthetic, like what you would get at the dentist, was administered around the site. To Robert's amazement, the patient didn't flinch (maybe he had a high pain tolerance after

224

all). The podiatry intern prepped the site with an alcohol-based product and then draped it.

Next, the podiatry intern, who was a hairy, slightly overweight, 30-year-old man from Iowa, took a #15 blade and plunged it into the middle of the hemorrhoid … except this wasn't a hemorrhoid, and there was an immediate explosion. A combination of pus and feces under pressure shot out of the patient's perineum and onto the interns' heads, hitting Robert in the face and shirt. The podiatry intern took most of the explosion on his neck, and it ran down his hairy chest as a clot. There was at least 100 mL of purulent drainage—enough to fill a soda bottle—and a horrific smell of infection and old feces.

Literally covered in pus and shit, Robert and the intern paged the colorectal attending back to the room. The colorectal surgeon came in and said, "That's what I thought." The patient was then booked for surgery, Robert and the other intern looked at each other knowing they'd been set up by the attending surgeon.

Robert and the intern hit the showers, (the intern went home after that shift and shaved his chest!) and Robert went to the operating room for this disgusting case—nothing like debridement of these gangrene and fistula sites. After removing infected, necrotic tissue and more drainage, a washout was performed. Plastic surgery was consulted, and the patient was placed in a wound vac. (This VAC—vacuum-assisted closure—device pulls out drainage, allowing granular tissue to grow for healing.)

The patient was going to need skin grafts and was at risk for dysfunction of his rectum long term. Thankfully, he kept coming in for help. A true case of "rectum, damn near killed 'em!"

CHAPTER 43
Veterinary Medicine

Samantha was covering the surgery rotation and working with the bariatric surgeons. Many patients came in with other clinical conditions, infections, and trauma that were found to have morbid obesity. On service she was seeing patients with comorbidities typically seen in patients greater than 70 years of age, but they were in their 20s. The interns were also seeing advancing arthritis from this obesity.

Unfortunately, the hospital system lost its affiliation with one of the local colleges that had a veterinarian medicine school that worked with both small and large farm animals. Whenever a patient came in that was over 400 pounds, the doctors relied on the veterinarian school for any imaging. Simply put, the hospital's machines could not withstand the weight of the patients, nor could the patients fit within the circular CT or MRI scanners.

On rounds, the overnight team handed off a report to Samantha of a woman named Martha Lynn who had been transferred from an outlying hospital in the countryside to the trauma center because the hospital offered bariatric surgery. The smaller hospital had attempted a more minimally invasive bariatric procedure that was going wrong for the patient. Martha Lynn was a pleasant 580-pound southern belle who spent more than an hour putting on makeup in the morning. She wore a nightgown that could've been put on a horse, and she couldn't reach all the parts of her body to bathe. A musky smell came from her room, and she had significant edema to her extremities.

The attending bariatric surgeon instructed our service that the patient needed an MRI and that this would be set up with the veterinary school. When Samantha called to set this up and put the order in, she realized the contract had been lost. The veterinary school was no longer willing to take on the legal risk of imaging the patients. The doctors had worked out a deal where the images could be read by a radiologist; they just needed the disk to be transported.

Samantha wondered how they could help this patient as she was not healthy enough to have an exploratory surgery, and there was concern that the patient had infection at the previous site that had not turned septic. There was also concern that her immune system was not responding to the infection, and she was a ticking time bomb for a life-threatening illness.

Samantha had grown up in the country in the Midwest, the child of two factory workers, which made her not only understand the mentality of the patient, but she also had an unbelievable conscientiousness, tolerance to stress, and intellect. She figured that there would be some way to get this patient scanned, even if she had to convince the veterinary clinic to give her another chance.

Then the lightbulb went off in Samantha's mind. She had heard in the past that patients like these at other facilities could coordinate with local zoos to have imaging performed. She reached out to the administration at the local zoo and found they were more than willing to take on the patient. This had to be coordinated with the hospital administration, but it was actually a better rate than the veterinary school, so administration was all for this. This one lightbulb thought changed the way that imaging is done for these obese patients to date.

Samantha got to go with the patient as special transport was performed. (Fortunately, a company has developed an air-transport system that slides underneath the patient like a sheet and inflates so that the patient can be easily moved. As you can imagine, even two strong younger patient assistants or EMS providers that are former athletes could not move someone this large.) The patient was put in the special ambulance and driven to the local zoo.

When they arrived, they realized there was a problem. There was no way to get the patient out of the ambulance and onto the loading dock to bring her into the imaging center. At that point, they decided to use a forklift driven by one of the zoo operators. The patient agreed and signed a waiver, and they used the forklift to transfer her to the loading dock. Staying on the specialized bed constructed for someone of her weight, she was lifted onto the dock and wheeled into the MRI.

The zoo had just finished working to get an MRI of an elephant and had the setup for the patient. Somehow, through all this, Martha Lynn seemed unfazed. Perhaps she was in such a deep depression that she didn't even recognize that she was using an elephant MRI for imaging. Samantha could not wrap her head around this, thinking, *At what point do you tip the scale where you've eaten too much or your metabolism is slowed, and you can't help yourself anymore?*

On previous surgery rotations, Samantha had seen patients underestimate their weight by 100 to 150 pounds. This was common. They told the pre-surgical testing staff that they weighed 280 pounds, but when they showed up for surgery, they actually weighed 400 pounds.

These are tough conversations to have with patients, and it's difficult to see people hurt themselves in this way. It's truly a societal epidemic, and these folks need help from a mental healthcare standpoint. For these patients the day always comes when they become too weak that they can no longer get out of bed; it's a downward spiral from here, taking a toll not only on the whole-body system, but also a social and economic toll on the healthcare system at large.

ABOUT THE AUTHOR

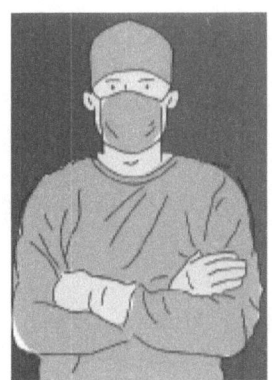

Dr. Brandon Green is a pseudonym for
the author, who wishes to remain
anonymous. The author is an Attending
Surgeon at a large city Level 1 Trauma
Center. The surgeon teaches residents
and fellows, is involved in research and
publications, and speaks at medical
conferences.

The short stories are real occurrences that happened to the
three interns in one residency year. The names and locations
have been changed to provide privacy protection and follow
HIPPA guidelines. The author recommends healthcare
workers process what they are experiencing by discussing
their own experiences from behind the scenes, as these
experiences. are likely happening at all hospitals throughout
the United States.

This is a work of sociology, psychology, medicine, surgery,
dealing with the public, putting others in front of yourself, and
self-reflective learning.

Thank you for taking the time to read and understand what's happening in modern society and healthcare training.